DEDICATION

This book is dedicated to my dear friend Pat Clutter, who set the example for me to be willing to take the risks to follow my dreams and "think outside the box". Pat has not only set the example, but has been kind enough to share leads and opportunities for me to be able to follow my own dreams. Pat has bravely followed me on crazy adventures not only in nursing but all around the world. Her companion-ship, mentorship, and friendship have helped shape me into the emergency nurse I am today.

Thanks Pat!

D1475981

To order additional copies of this book, or to see other products by Solheim Enterprises / Media Room E, please visit our easy to use store website:

SolheimEnterprises.com/products

To join the study group and get free CEN Exam advice and practice, like us on facebook at:

Facebook.com/ConferenceRoomE

Please send comments and suggestions to :

Jeff@solheimenterprises.com

To find a class near you, see our online calendar at:

SolheimEnterprises.com/calendar

Titles currently available at the SolheimEnterprises.com store:

For the **CEN Exam,** by Jeff Solheim

 CEN Pocket Practice Books, 2nd edition—each pocket size book has hundreds of practice questions with answers and rationales. Each book covers different topics on the CEN Exam.

 CEN Pocket Pearls Books, 2nd edition—each pocket size book includes hundreds of Jeff Solheim's 'pearls of wisdom' for emergency nurses.

CEN Exam Review Course Manual—you can now order the actual course manual Jeff wrote and uses to teach his CEN Exam review course.

For the CCRN Exam, by Cammy House-Fancher

 CCRN Pocket Practice Books—each pocket size book has hundreds of practice questions with answers and rationales. Each book covers different topics on the CCRN Exam.

Coming soon…

Pocket Practice books for the **CPEN Exam,** by Cathy Fox and Melissa Weir

Course Manuals for the **CCRN Exam,** and **CPEN Exam**

Author's Note

I suspect that many people will use this pocket book as a study guide to prepare to take the Certification in Emergency Nursing Exam (CEN)® . I am certain this can be a valuable tool for that goal. I highly recommend that the pocket books be used to <u>augment</u> preparation for the exam. These books were not written or designed as the sole tool for studying. They should instead be used to re-enforce and solidify knowledge gained from more complete sources. The "pearls of wisdom" within this book may sometimes contain concepts or words that the reader may be unfamiliar with. Seize that opportunity to seek out more information about the concept or word so that the "pearl" makes sense. By doing that, the reader can maximize their learning potential. Good luck in your endeavors.

Jeff Solheim

Table of contents

Gastroin-
testinal
Disorders

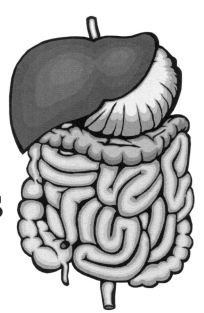

ⓟ When gastric contents regurgitate from the stomach into the esophagus, it is termed gastroesophageal reflux disease (GERD).

ⓟ Mallory-Weiss tears are defined as small tears in the blood vessels at the junction of the esophagus and stomach. They are caused by violent retching or vomiting.

ⓟ Common precipitants to the development of esophageal varices are alcoholism and cirrhosis of the liver.

ⓟ An inflammation of the lining of the stomach is called gastritits.

ⓟ The optimal position for inserting a gastric tube in the obtunded patient is head of bed down, preferably on the left side.

ⓟ Blood in the stool which cannot be detected with the naked eye is termed occult blood.

ⓟ Hepatitis A is easily spread through fecal contamination and oral ingestion and is more common in the developing world where overcrowded conditions exist and sanitation is difficult to maintain.

- Ⓟ Esophagitis is an inflammation of the mucosa of the esophagus.
- Ⓟ Common causes of acute pancreatitis are obstructions in the bile duct or ingestion of excessive alcohol.
- Ⓟ Infections from Hepatitis A are generally mild, acute and short-lived.
- Ⓟ Risk factors for gastroesophageal reflux disease include obesity, pregnancy and passing the age of 40.
- Ⓟ The constant irritation of the esophagus caused by the acid reflux of gastroesophageal reflux disorder can ultimately contribute to esophagitis.
- Ⓟ The most common esophageal obstruction is either a food bolus or a bone in the adult.
- Ⓟ Engorged blood vessels in the lower esophagus and upper stomach are referred to as esophageal varices.
- Ⓟ Helicobacter pylori is a gram-negative bacterium that thrives in the lining of the stomach, leading to irritation, gastritis and ulcers.

Ⓟ Duodenal ulcers are most common between the ages of 30 and 55 years of age.

Ⓟ Gastric ulcers are most common between the ages of 55 and 70 years of age.

Ⓟ Hepatitis B may be spread parenterally, sexually, through perinatal transmission, human bites, and permucosal exposure to blood or blood products.

Ⓟ The classic sign of cholecystitis is sudden onset right upper quadrant or epigastric pain that may be referred to the right scapula and shoulder or around the right side to the supraclavicular area.

Ⓟ Non-inflammatory diarrhea, caused by agents such as *C. difficile, Giardia lamblia*, and *E. Coli* prevent the colon from absorbing water, resulting in watery diarrhea.

Ⓟ Inflammatory diarrhea, caused by the rotavirus, Norwalk virus, *S. dysenteriae, Salmonella, E. coli* and *Campyobacter jejuni* results in bloody diarrhea and fever.

- Ⓟ The classic sign of peritonitis is severe abdominal pain which is exacerbated by movement or coughing.
- Ⓟ Food poisoning can be differentiated from other forms of diarrhea because it usually affects numerous people and is marked by vomiting as well as diarrhea.
- Ⓟ Diverticulitis is inflammation of diverticula.
- Ⓟ Diverticula are pouches in the bowel wall.
- Ⓟ Colitis is an inflammation of the colon that results in ulcers of the mucosa of the colon.
- Ⓟ Regional ileitis is also known as Crohn's disease.
- Ⓟ Complications of bowel obstructions may include dehydration, bowel ischemia, and bowel perforation.
- Ⓟ Pyloric stenosis is marked by hypertrophy and hyperplasia of the pylorus muscle and narrowing of the gastric antrum.
- Ⓟ Hepatitis B can be acute or chronic. Chronic cases go on to cause liver cirrhosis, liver failure, and liver cancer.

Ⓟ The stomach is more frequently injured in penetrating as opposed to blunt trauma.

Ⓟ A hiatal hernia is a condition where the upper part of the stomach herniates through the opening in the diaphragm through which the esophagus passes.

Ⓟ Pediatric patients have greater fluid needs related to body surface area, therefore mild cases of nausea, vomiting and diarrhea can lead to profound illness in the pediatric patient.

Ⓟ Clay colored stools are an indication of a blocked bile duct or failing liver.

Ⓟ Certain infections, such as the mumps, coxsackie virus, hepatits B virus, *Mycoplasma* sp., *Legionalla* sp., and ascariasis have been known to cause acute pancreatitis.

Ⓟ The pain of cholecystitis may be aggravated by taking a deep breath and often follows ingestion of a large meal as well as fried or fatty foods.

- Ⓟ Pain in early appendicitis may be in the periumbilical region before settling into the right lower quadrant.
- Ⓟ Patients who consume a low fiber diet have a higher incidence of diverticulitis.
- Ⓟ The majority of pyloric stenosis occurs between the third and twelfth week of life.
- Ⓟ Hepatitis C may be spread through parenteral means, permucosal exposure to blood or blood products, high risk sexual contact, or perinatal contact.
- Ⓟ The most common site of inflammation in regional ileitis is the ileum, although in severe cases it may spread anywhere between the esophagus to the rectum.
- Ⓟ Hepatitis C frequently results in chronic infections. It may be asymptomatic at first and clinical manifestations may not appear until the disease has progressed and liver failure has started.
- Ⓟ The stomach of children is more frequently injured then their adult counterparts.

- ℗ The symptoms of food poisoning typically occur 4 – 6 hours after ingestion of the causative agent.
- ℗ Hepatitis D is a unique form of hepatitis that requires Hepatitis B for replication and survival, therefore patients with Hepatitis D will always have hepatitis B.
- ℗ A bowel obstruction with no bowel movements likely indicates a complete obstruction; a bowel obstruction with diarrhea likely indicates a partial bowel obstruction.
- ℗ Parents should be taught not to give apple juice to dehydrated infants, as this is hyperosmolar and can worsen diarrhea.
- ℗ The pain of esophageal reflux disease is often described as a burning sensation that moves up and down the chest and may radiate to the neck, shoulders, arm, back or abdomen.
- ℗ Achalasia is impaired motility of the lower two thirds of the esophagus and can lead to esophagitis.
- ℗ Ruptured esophageal varices can result in rapid and life-threatening blood loss.

- ⓟ Ingestion of noxious substances such as NSAIDs, alcohol, salicylates, steroids, acids, alkalis or foods with excessive seasoning can cause or exacerbate gastritis.
- ⓟ To estimate the length of a gastric tube, measure the distance from the tip of the nose to the earlobe and down to the xiphoid process.
- ⓟ Possible causes of pancreatitis include hypercalcemia, hyperlipidemia, scorpion bites, organophosphate insecticides and trauma to the pancreas.
- ⓟ One sign of cholecystitis is the inability to take a deep breath when palpating under the right upper quadrant (Murphy's sign).
- ⓟ The symptoms of hepatitis B and hepatitis D are similar, but patients infected with both carry a much higher risk for cirrhosis.
- ⓟ Pressure on the left lower abdomen may intensify pain in the right lower quadrant (Rovsing's sign) in patients with appendicitis.
- ⓟ The two most common causes of liver cirrhosis is alcoholism and hepatitis C.

- Ⓟ Serum ammonia levels are usually high with liver cirrhosis and may contribute to hepatic encephalopathy which is marked by confusion.
- Ⓟ Patients with peritonitis may find that flexing the knees decreases their discomfort.
- Ⓟ Regional ileitis is more common amongst smokers.
- Ⓟ The symptoms of a small bowel obstruction typically develop more quickly than a large bowel obstruction.
- Ⓟ Intussusception is a condition where the bowel telescopes on itself.
- Ⓟ Symptoms of a hiatal hernia are worse when the patient coughs, bends forward, wears tight clothing, has ascites, is obese, pregnant or supine.
- Ⓟ Blunt trauma to the diaphragmatic area, such as a kick to the upper abdomen or being propelled into the handlebars of a bicycle are associated with pancreatic trauma.

- Ⓟ Hepatitis E is contracted from drinking water contaminated with the virus or eating fish who have been in contaminated water.
- Ⓟ The pain of esophageal reflux disease often initiates with activities that increase intra-abdominal pressure such as lifting, straining, or assuming the recumbent position.
- Ⓟ Infections of the esophagus from conditions such as *Candida*, herpes simplex, and cytomegalovirus can lead to esophagitis.
- Ⓟ Consumption of excessive food or alcohol may cause a rupture of the esophageal wall. This is known as Boerhaave's syndrome.
- Ⓟ Factors which can cause esophageal varices to rupture includes sneezing, coughing, straining at stool, lifting heavy objects, vomiting, or swallowing poorly chewed foods.
- Ⓟ Chronic pancreatitis degrades the organs' ability to digest protein, carbohydrates and fats.
- Ⓟ The classic pain of pancreatitis is a sharp boring pain in the epigastric region which radiates through to the back.

(P) Jaundice is one indication of a blocked bile duct.

(P) Liver dysfunction will result in decreased production of albumin. Decreased serum albumin will cause fluid to shift out of the vasculature resulting in peripheral edema and ascites.

(P) Common sources of food poisoning are raw or inadequately cooked shrimp, shellfish or meat.

(P) There is no cure for hepatitis. Acute cases must run their course. The severity of chronic cases may be diminished with interferons and ribavirin.

(P) Findings with peritonitis include diffuse abdominal pain and a rigid abdomen, fever, tenderness to palpation and rebound tenderness.

(P) The pain of diverticulitis is usually an abrupt onset of aching cramping pain that may be generalized but usually settles into the left lower quadrant.

(P) Hiatal hernias contribute to gastroesophageal reflux disorder and esophagitis.

Ⓟ Indications of stomach trauma include left upper quadrant pain, surface trauma to the left chest or left upper quadrant, hematemesis, decreased bowel sounds and a rigid abdomen.

Ⓟ Parents should be taught to give infants and children with dehydration glucose water, pediatric electrolyte drinks, broth, Jell-O, Kool-Aid, tea or popsicles.

Ⓟ Patients with Mallory-Weiss tears will usually present with varying degrees of bloody emesis.

Ⓟ Ulcer pain is usually epigastric and may radiate through to the mid-back. It may be described as "squeezing", "indigestion", "gnawing", "colicky", "aching" or "feeling of fullness".

Ⓟ Things which can exacerbate the pain of pancreatitis include eating, alcohol intake, walking or lying supine.

Ⓟ Intussusception in adults commonly occurs near a colon tumor or polyp.

ⓟ Patients with pancreatitis may find that their pain is relieved by leaning forward or assuming the fetal position.

ⓟ Palpating the abdomen of a patient with diverticulitis will usually reveal tenderness and guarding to the left lower quadrant.

ⓟ Symptoms found in both ulcerative colitis **AND** regional ileitis includes abdominal distension, anemia, weight loss, low grade fever, nausea, vomiting, abdominal cramping and distension.

ⓟ Vomiting is a more common finding with small bowel obstructions than large bowel obstructions.

ⓟ Clinical manifestations of pyloric stenosis include poor weight gain, continual hunger, jaundice, and gastric peristalsis prior to emesis.

ⓟ The most common location for an intussesception is the near the ileocecal valve or a Merkel's diverticulum in children.

ⓟ Ulcerative colitis tends to inflame the mucosal layer of the bowel, regional ileitis may inflame all layers of the bowel.

- Ⓟ The spleen is the most commonly injured abdominal organ in blunt trauma.
- Ⓟ Perforations of hollow organs such as the stomach cause free air on an x-ray.
- Ⓟ The pain of gastroesophageal reflux disorder is usually most acute 30 – 60 minutes after eating.
- Ⓟ Cholinergic drugs such as Bethanechol (Urecholine) are given to increase lower esophageal sphincter pressure, facilitating gastric emptying.
- Ⓟ Patients with Boerhaave's syndrome will usually present with significant bloody emesis and severe retrosternal chest pain.
- Ⓟ Ingesting irritating fluids, salicylates or drugs may cause esophageal varices to start bleeding.
- Ⓟ If Benzocaine, tetracaine, or lidocaine is sprayed into the nose prior to gastric tube insertion, spraying time should not exceed two seconds to prevent systemic effects of these drugs.

Ⓟ Duodenal ulcers are usually more painful before meals and are relieved by food or antacids.

Ⓟ The pain of gastric ulcers is more likely to be worse after meals.

Ⓟ Orogastric tubes, rather than nasogastric tubes should be placed on
   all patients with suspected head injuries or basilar skull fractures.

Ⓟ Palpating the abdomen of a patient with pancreatitis will usually
   reveal tenderness.

Ⓟ Abnormal lab values associated with cholecystitis include elevated
   white blood cell counts, increased serum and urine bilirubin levels,
   and increased alanine aminotransferase (ALT).

Ⓟ Diarrhea without nausea should be treated with oral rehydration
   agents such as electrolyte "sports drink", colas, ginger ale, apple
   juice, tea or broth.

Ⓟ Patients with regional ileitis often have 3 – 4 semi formed stools a
   day that are foul smelling and may contain undigested fat.

- Ⓟ Early symptoms of small bowel obstructions include vomiting undigested food. As the obstruction progresses, the patient may vomit bile and fecal material.
- Ⓟ Most volvulus occurs in children prior to the age of one, with many occurring prior to the first month of life. As many as 25% or more occur in the first week of life.
- Ⓟ Fractures of ribs 10 through 12 on the left side are associated with splenic trauma.
- Ⓟ Although rarely injured, trauma to the pancreas carries a high mortality because it is often a missed injury.
- Ⓟ Patients with esophageal reflux disorder may complain of painful swallowing (odynophagia) or difficulty swallowing (dysphagia) especially when supine.
- Ⓟ The verbal adult with an esophageal obstruction will usually present to the ED with complaints of difficulty swallowing and pain in the chest around the area of the obstruction.

Ⓟ Treatment for bleeding esophageal varices revolves around treating hypovolemic shock and controlling bleeding.

Ⓟ Physical or emotional stress, tobacco, radiation, bacterial or viral infection or *helicobacter pylori* infection are all causes of gastritis or may exacerbate pre-existing gastritis.

Ⓟ Hematemesis is bloody emesis.

Ⓟ Hematochezia is bright red blood in the stool.

Ⓟ Melena is dark, black, sticky stool associated with partially digested blood in the gastrointestinal tract.

Ⓟ Jaundice is first noticed on elastic body tissues such as the sclera and palate, followed by the palms of the hands and the soles of the feet.

Ⓟ Common lab values associated with pancreatitis include an elevated white blood cell count, elevated serum amylase and lipase and elevated glucose levels.

- Ⓟ Patients with decreased serum albumin will usually have decreased serum calcium.
- Ⓟ Patients with liver dysfunction will produce less clotting factors resulting in symptoms such as easy bruising and increased incidence of bleeding.
- Ⓟ Common problems associated with severe diarrhea include metabolic acidosis, potassium, glucose and calcium abnormalities.
- Ⓟ Patients with appendicitis will often find that flexing the knees decreases abdominal pain.
- Ⓟ Patients with diverticulitis often have a low grade fever, an elevated white count with a shift to the left and occult blood in the stool.
- Ⓟ Patients with ulcerative colitis tend to have 5 – 25 stools per day containing blood, fat and pus and may experience rectal bleeding.
- Ⓟ The pain of a small bowel obstruction is described as crampy and intermittent. The pain of large bowel obstructions is more often described as a sensation of fullness and more low-grade.

Ⓟ A mobile, hard, olive shaped mass may be palpated over the pyloris in pyloric stenosis.

Ⓟ Indications of splenic trauma include left upper quadrant pain which may radiate to the left shoulder as well as signs of hypo-volemia.

Ⓟ The pain of pancreatic trauma may not occur until several hours after the event, but will ultimately result in epigastric pain.

Ⓟ Water brash is defined as regurgitation of an excessive accumula-tion of saliva from the lower part of the esophagus, often with some acid material from the stomach.

Ⓟ Dopamine antagonist such as Metoclopramide (Reglan) are given to move food through the digestive system faster.

Ⓟ Vasoconstrictive agents such as vasopressin (Pitressin) or san-dostatin (Octreotide) may be given to control gastrointestinal bleeding.

Ⓟ Patients with gastritis often find that food will diminish their pain.

- Ⓟ Placement of gastric tubes in patients with esophageal varices carries a risk of rupturing a varices and causing hemorrhage.
- Ⓟ Patients with severe pancreatitis may develop hypocalcemia.
- Ⓟ Antibiotics are prescribed for diarrhea caused by bacteria, and corticosteroids may be prescribed for parasitical diarrhea.
- Ⓟ Inflammatory changes associated with pancreatitis may lead to pleural effusions, and the development of acute respiratory distress syndrome.
- Ⓟ Helicobacter pylori is transmitted either through the fecal-oral route, tainted water supplies or through the saliva of one infected individual to another.
- Ⓟ Pancreatitis can cause pancreatic juices to leak into the abdomen, causing intra-abdominal bleeding and hypovolemia.
- Ⓟ Pain that increases when pressure is relieved while palpating is termed rebound tenderness and is an indication of peritoneal irritation.

- Ⓟ An inguinal hernia is a condition where intestinal contents protrude through the inguinal canal.
- Ⓟ Indications of pancreatic trauma include abdominal distension, diminished bowel sounds, tenderness to palpation and abdominal rigidity, especially in the epigastric region.
- Ⓟ Patients with esophageal reflux disorder may describe symptoms such as regurgitation, belching, nausea, anorexia, weight loss, loss of dental enamel, bad breath and hoarseness.
- Ⓟ Antacids such as Maalox will neutralize acids in the stomach.
- Ⓟ Histamine H_2-receptor antagonists such as Ranitidine (Zantac) are given to block acid production.
- Ⓟ Proton pump inhibitors such as Lansoprazole (Prevacid) are given to shut down acid pumps in the stomach and reduce acidity.
- Ⓟ Patients infected with fecal-oral hepatitis (hepatitis A and E) should be taught to avoid handling foods that will be eaten by others, to use a private bathroom and to avoid alcohol consumption.

- Ⓟ Acid protective agents such as Sucralfate (Carafate) provide a thick protective coat over the lower esophagus and stomach to protect it from excess acidity.
- Ⓟ Hepatitis E is uncommon in the United States, and is more commonly found in Asia, Africa and Mexico.
- Ⓟ Fractures of ribs 8 through 12 on the right side are associated with liver trauma.
- Ⓟ Bruising of the flanks (Grey-Turner's sign) is one indication of hemorrhagic pancreatitis.
- Ⓟ Liver infection from the hepatitis E virus is usually mild and short-lived and rarely becomes chronic or life threatening.
- Ⓟ Patients with flare-ups of regional ileitis or ulcerative colitis will often present with complaints of extreme pain and dehydration.
- Ⓟ Large bowel obstructions result in severe abdominal distension, but this is less common with small bowel obstructions.
- Ⓟ Bruising around the umbilicus (Cullen's sign) is one indication of hemorrhagic pancreatitis.

Ⓟ Common signs of hepatitis include abdominal pain, anorexia, nausea and vomiting, joint pain, hepatomegaly and occasionally splenomegaly.

Ⓟ Common pharmacological agents used to control regional ileitis and ulcerative colitis include anticholinergics, antidiarrheals, anti-inflammatories, antimicrobials, and corticosteroids.

Ⓟ The most common age for intussusception to occur is between the ages of 3 months and one year.

Ⓟ Hepatitis infections that last less than six months are considered acute and those that last longer than six months are termed chronic.

Ⓟ Serum amylase, lipase and glucose may elevate after pancreatic trauma, although this may take up to six hours to develop.

Ⓟ Discharge teaching for gastroesophageal reflux disorder should include avoidance of fatty foods, chocolate, peppermint and spearmint, tea, coffee, onions, garlic and alcohol.

- ℗ Fluid replacement in the dehydrated child is given at 20 mL/kg.
- ℗ When administering vasopressin (Pitressin) or sandostatin (Octreotide), monitor for hypertension.
- ℗ Symptoms of gastritis include epigastric pain, nausea and vomiting, diarrhea, anorexia and flatulence.
- ℗ Patients with pancreatitis may develop abscesses and sepsis. They should be monitored for increasing fever, increasing abdominal pain or indications of sepsis.
- ℗ Treatment for diverticulitis may include "nothing by mouth" status, insertion of a gastric tube, anticholinergics, IV fluid replacement, and antibiotic therapy.
- ℗ Lab values found in hepatitis include elevated liver enzymes, leukopenia, increased lymphocyte counts, positive hepatitis antibody/antigen screen and prolonged prothrombin time.
- ℗ Immunosuppressants such as Mercaptopurine [Purinethol] or Azathioprine [Imuran] may be used to treat ulcerative colitis or regional ileitis.

Ⓟ Auscultation may reveal high-pitched peristaltic rush sounds proximal to the area of the an intestinal obstruction.

Ⓟ A driver's spleen is frequently injured when there is a side impact collision on the driver's side of the vehicle.

Ⓟ The inability of the liver to dump bilirubin into the intestines because of hepatitis may cause clay-colored stools, dark frothy urine and the development of jaundice.

Ⓟ Intussusception is marked by colicky pain associated with peristalsis. The child may rest for 15 – 30 minutes, then cry with pain and pull legs to abdomen for 15-30 minutes, then fall back asleep.

Ⓟ Dehydrated children may not have alterations in blood pressure until they have lost 25% of their fluids, therefore tachycardia, poor skin turgor, and sunken fontanelles should be assessed for.

Ⓟ Long-term use of drugs which irritate the esophagus such as NSAIDs, potassium chloride, quinidine and antibiotics can lead to esophagitis.

Ⓟ Patients with hepatitis should be encouraged to increase their calorie intake, and consume a diet of small, frequent feedings low in fat and high in carbohydrates.

Ⓟ Recent ingestion of red meat can give false positive tests when using a hemoccult testing card and solution.

Ⓟ Dark colored urine that foams when shaken is indicative of high serum bilirubin levels and probable blockage of the common bile duct.

Ⓟ The pain of pancreatitis may be severe and require significant analgesia.

Ⓟ Appendicitis is usually marked by a white blood cell count above 10,000 cells/mm^3 with increased neutrophils – especially immature neutrophils called "bands".

Ⓟ Foods which tend to exacerbate regional ileitis and colitis include raw fruits and vegetables as well as fatty or spicy foods.

Ⓟ Pancreatic trauma usually requires surgical intervention.

Ⓟ Early bowel obstructions may cause borborygmi (hyperactive bowel sounds) early on which progresses to absent bowel sounds in later phases.

Ⓟ Stool which look like grape jelly may be an indication of intussusception.

Ⓟ The small bowel (duodenum, jejunum, and ileum) is more frequently injured in trauma because it is more central and exposed in the abdomen then the large bowel.

Ⓟ The most commonly injured areas of the large bowel are the transverse and sigmoid colon.

Ⓟ The abdominal contents are less protected in pediatric patients therefore, trauma to abdominal organs is more common in this age group.

Ⓟ Medications known to exacerbate gastroesophageal reflux disorder include nitrates, calcium channel blockers, nicotine, caffeine, anticholinergics, theophylline, and diazepam (Valium).

Ⓟ Vaccines exist to prevent infections from Hepatitis A and B.

Ⓟ Nitroglycerin may be given with vasopressin (Pitressin) or sandostatin (Octreotide) to prevent myocardial ischemia.

Ⓟ Nitroglycerin or papaverine are used to relax smooth muscles and reduce the discomfort of pancreatitis.

Ⓟ Pharmacological agents used to treat severe diarrhea include antiemetics, analgesics, and anticholingergics.

Ⓟ Abdominal ultrasound and computerized tomography may be used to diagnose appendicitis.

Ⓟ Patients with regional ileitis and ulcerative colitis should be taught to avoid drinking fluids with meals to prevent intestinal distension.

Ⓟ Patients with volvulus exhibit abdominal distension, vomiting and progressively worsening pain.

Ⓟ Antispasmodics such as dicyclomine (Bentyl) or propantheline bromide (Pro-Banthine) – decrease vagal stimulation and release of pancreatic enzymes in pancreatitis.

- Ⓟ One potential complication of regional ileitis is fistulas that form between loops of bowel. Fistulas may also develop between the bowel and the vagina, bladder or skin.
- Ⓟ Men get inguinal hernias more often than women.
- Ⓟ Bowel injuries may have little symptoms and not manifest until peritonitis from peritoneal contamination becomes evident.
- Ⓟ An indication of an esophageal obstruction in a pediatric patient includes dysphagia, drooling, vomiting, gagging and anorexia.
- Ⓟ Endoscopy may be used to control gastrointestinal bleeding.
- Ⓟ When a gastric tube reaches the pharynx during insertion, have the patient flex the head forward to close off the upper airway but leave the esophagus open.
- Ⓟ Carbonic anhydrase inhibitors, such as acetazolamide (Diamox) ,are used to reduce volume and concentration of pancreatic secretions in pancreatitis.

- Ⓟ Treatment for appendicitis includes "nothing by mouth", IV access, analgesics, antipyretics, antiemetics and possible gastric tube.
- Ⓟ A common complication of peritonitis is dehydration and electrolyte imbalances.
- Ⓟ Patients with regional ileitis or colitis may suffer malnutrition due to malabsorption of nutrients. Nutritional supplements may be required.
- Ⓟ Antacids are used to neutralize gastric secretions which in turn decreases pancreatic secretions in pancreatitis.
- Ⓟ Signs of bowel injury include generalized abdominal pain, nausea and vomiting, hypovolemia, sepsis, diminished or absent bowel sounds, rebound tenderness and abdominal rigidity.
- Ⓟ Beta-adrenergic blockers, progesterone and estrogen are known to exacerbate gastroesophageal reflux disorders.
- Ⓟ A Sengstaken-Blakemore tube or Minnesota tube may be utilized to temporarily stem the bleeding of esophageal varices.

ⓟ Most cases of Mallory-Weiss tears require no treatment. If bleeding is severe, endoscopy with injection of epinephrine into the bleeding vessels may be required.

ⓟ Drugs that reduce stomach acidity are used to treat gastritis.

ⓟ Nasogastric tubes should not be placed in infants because they are obligatory nose breathers. Orogastric tubes may be placed.

ⓟ Histamine H_2-receptor antagonists such as cimetidine (Tagamet) and ranitidine (Zantac) may decrease hydrochloric acid which can diminish pancreatic secretions in pancreatitis.

ⓟ A severe complication of regional ileitis or ulcerative colitis is toxic megacolon, a dilation of the bowel that may lead to perforation.

ⓟ Manifestations of toxic megacolon include abdominal tenderness, loss of bowel sounds, colonic dilation on abdominal film, an elevated white blood cell count and indications of sepsis.

ⓟ Most bowel injuries require surgical intervention.

Ⓟ A frequent cause of death in pediatric maltreatment cases is abdominal trauma.

Ⓟ Glucagon, a smooth muscle relaxant, may be used to treat esophageal obstructions.

Ⓟ A Sengstaken-Blakemore tube or Minnesota tube has gastric and esophageal balloons that can be inflated to put pressure on the lower esophagus and upper stomach to reduce bleeding.

Ⓟ Discharge instructions for patients being discharged home with an ulcer include consumption of a bland low-fiber diet, decreased stress and avoidance of salicylates.

Ⓟ Radishes, turnips, cabbage, cauliflower, horseradish, uncooked broccoli, and cantaloupe contain a chemical which can give a false positive when using a hemoccult testing card and solution.

Ⓟ When the bile duct is blocked, patients may complain of feeling nauseated, anorexic, or feeling full after eating fatty foods because the liver does not secrete enzymes to digest fats.

- ⓟ Treatment for cholecystitis includes initiation of intravenous fluids, antiemetics, and maintenance of nothing by mouth (NPO) status.
- ⓟ Patients with severe watery diarrhea should be encouraged to maintain a clear liquid diet and remain hydrated.
- ⓟ Pregnant patients with appendicitis may have pain in the right upper quadrant.
- ⓟ Accumulation of abdominal fluid in peritonitis may push the diaphragm upwards resulting in respiratory difficulties.
- ⓟ When discharging a patient home with diverticulitis, encourage the patient to drink at least eight glasses of water daily, to use stool softeners and avoid straining while defecating.
- ⓟ When palpating the abdomen of a patient with intussusception, a palpable sausage shaped mass may be noted in the right lower or middle abdomen over the intussusceptions site.
- ⓟ Reduction of an inguinal hernia involves administering analgesia, placing the patient in the Trendelenberg's position, and applying ice to the area.

- Ⓟ A Focused Assessment Sonography for Trauma (FAST) is a bedside ultrasound often employed to detect bleeding in the abdomen, chest, pelvis or pericardial sac.
- Ⓟ The symptoms of gastroesophageal reflux disorder and esophagitis are similar except esophagitis usually causes more constant discomfort.
- Ⓟ Glucagon may be used to reduce pancreatic inflammation and decreases serum amylase as well as suppress pancreatic secretions in pancreatitis.
- Ⓟ Findings associated with bowel obstructions include fever, indications of severe dehydration, elevated white blood cell counts, diffuse abdominal tenderness and rigidity.
- Ⓟ Indications of liver trauma include right upper quadrant pain that may radiate to the right shoulder, a rigid abdomen with possible rebound tenderness and hypovolemic shock.
- Ⓟ Esophagoscopy may be used to retrieve esophageal obstructions.
- Ⓟ A common finding in patients with liver dysfunction is anemia.

- ℗ Potential risk factors associated with a Sengstaken-Blakemore tube or Minnesota tube includes gastric or esophageal perforation as well as ischemia around the balloons.
- ℗ Helicobacter pylori is treated with antibiotics.
- ℗ One indication of gastrointestinal bleeding is an elevated blood urea nitrogen level without a similar increase in serum creatinine.
- ℗ Yellow, bulky, fatty appearing stools are termed steatorrhea and indicate a lack of bile salts in conditions such as pancreatitis or blocked bile ducts.
- ℗ Lactulose is used to decrease serum ammonia levels.
- ℗ Elderly people with appendicitis may lack fever and abdominal pain.
- ℗ NSAIDs, potassium chloride, quinidine and antibiotics, taken with inadequate fluid, may exacerbate esophagitis.
- ℗ Patients with bruising to the lower abdomen from a lap belt should be suspected of having intra-abdominal injuries and lumbar spinal fractures. This is called the "lap belt complex."

Ⓟ Somatostatin is used to inhibit pancreatic secretions in pancreatitis.

Ⓟ Patients with active diverticulitis should be encouraged to consume a low-fat, low fiber diet during the infection and a high fiber diet after resolution of the infection to prevent recurrence.

Ⓟ Discharge teaching for gastroesophageal reflux disorder should include eating small meals, elevating the head of the bed on 6 – 8 inch blocks, and stressing the importance of weight loss.

Ⓟ Treatment for Boerhaave's syndrome includes intravenous fluid replacement, administration of antibiotics and urgent surgical repair.

Ⓟ Severe cases of gastritis may require "nothing by mouth" status, and a gastric tube to empty and rest the stomach.

Ⓟ Surgical intervention is required for patients with a volvulus and pyloric stenosis.

Ⓟ Patients with peritonitis require surgical intervention. Analgesia, antiemetics, antibiotics and antipyretics may be given in the interim.

Ⓟ A barium enema may be used to reduce an intussusception.

Ⓟ Both the liver and spleen are highly vascular organs and trauma may to either may result in significant blood loss.

Ⓟ Citrus fruits and vitamin C supplements can give a false positive reading when using a hemoccult testing card and solution.

Ⓟ Analgesics are used in the treatment of cholecystitis. Antibiotics may also be given prophylactically to prevent infection.

Ⓟ Treatment for toxic megacolon involves intravenous rehydration, nothing by mouth (NPO) status and gastric tube to suction, antibiotic therapy, corticosteroids and surgical intervention.

Ⓟ Labs associated with pyloric stenosis include elevated bilirubin, hypochloremia, and hypokalemia.

Ⓟ Angiography can be used to identify active gastrointestinal bleeding and if a site of bleeding is noted with angiography, the site may be embolized, or a stent or coil used to stem the bleeding.

ⓟ Older adults are less likely to experience pain as they age and may have less acute presentations of abdominal emergencies.

ⓟ Treatment for bowel obstructions include intravenous fluid replacement, and "nothing by mouth" status.

ⓟ Indications of an inguinal hernia include a hernia which does not decrease in size when the patient is supine, elevated white blood cell count, rectal bleeding and signs of sepsis.

ⓟ Excessive use of tap water to irrigate a gastric tube can cause hyponatremia.

ⓟ Helicobacter pylori infection may be detected by a blood test.

ⓟ ⓟ The classic early sign of hepatitis is fatigue and malaise.

Bibliography for gastrointestinal emergencies

Bjerke, H. S. (2010, January 2). *Pancreatic trauma*. (E. Dunn, R. L. Sheriman, F. Talavera, P. Zamboni, & J. Geibel, Editors) Retrieved December 24, 2011, from emedicine.com: http://www.emedicine.com/med/topic2801.htm

Carter, J. S. (2004, November 2). *Atoms, molecules, water and pH*. Retrieved December 24, 2011, from File atom H_2O: http://biology.clc.uc.edu/courses/bio104/atom-h2o.htm

Corbett, J. V. (2004). *Laboratory tests and diagnostic procedures* (6 ed.). Upper Saddle River: Pearson Prentice Hall.

Danis, D., Blansfield, J., & Gervasini, A. (2007). *Handbook of clinical trauma: the first hour* (4 ed.). St. Louis: Mosby Elsevier.

Emergency Nurses Association. (2004). *Emergency Nursing Pediatric Course Provider Manual* (3 ed.). Des Plaines: Emergency Nurses Association.

Emergency Nurses Association. (2007). *Trauma Nursing Core Course Provider Manual* (6 ed.). Des Plaines Il: Emergency Nurses Association.

Hebra, A. (2011, October 5). *Intestinal volvulus*. Retrieved December 24, 2011, from eMedicine: http://www.emedicine.com/ped/topic1205.htm

Hoyt, K. S., & Selfridge-Thomas, J. (Eds.). (2007). *Emergency Nursing Core Curriculum* (6 ed.). St. Louis: Saunders Elsevier.

Kowalak, J. P., & Welsh, W. (Eds.). (2003). *Handbook of diagnostic tests* (3 ed.). Baltimore: Lippincott Williams and Wilkins.

Kunz Howard P, Steinmann, RA. (Eds.) (2010). Sheehy's Emergency Nursing: Principles and Practice. 6th ed. St. Louis: Mosby.

McCance, K. L., & Heuther, S. E. (2006). *Pathophysiology: The biologic basis for disease in adults and children (*5th ed.*).* St. Louis: Mosby.

Mower-Wade, D., & Kang, T. (2007). Can the spleen be saved? *Nursing 2007 Critical Care , 2* (4), 54-61.

Peitzman, A. B., Rhodes, M., Schwab, C. W., Yealy, D. M., & Fabian, T. C. (2007). *The trauma manual: trauma and acute care surgery.* Philadelphia : Lippincott Williams and Wilkins.

Proehl, J. (2009). *Emergency Nursing Procedures* (4 ed.). St. Louis: Saunders.

Ritchie, A. H., & Williscroft, D. M. (2006). Elevated liver enzymes as a predictor of liver injury in stable blunt abdominal trauma patients: case report and systematic review of the literature. *Can J Rural Med , 11* (4), 283 - 287.

Rooks, M. (2011, May 25). *Esophagus, foriegn body*. Retrieved December 24, 2011 from eMedicine: http://www.emedicine.com/radio/TOPIC272.HTM

Seth, D., Kamat, D., & Pansare, M. (2007). Foreign-Body Aspiration: A Guide to Early Detection. *Optimal Therapy in Consultant for Pediatrics* , *6* (1), 13 - 18.

GENITORUINARY EMERGENCIES

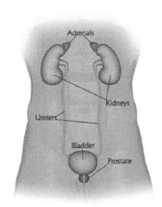

- Ⓟ Patients who contract Herpes type II will experience flu like symptoms shortly after exposure followed by stinging and burning around the genitalia and eruption of blisters near the pain.
- Ⓟ An infection of the urethra is termed urethritis.
- Ⓟ An infection of the bladder is termed cystitis.
- Ⓟ An infection of the ureters is termed ureteritis.
- Ⓟ An infection of the kidney is termed pyelonephritis.
- Ⓟ When teaching a patient how to collect a clean catch urine specimen, discourage them from stopping urine flow when positioning the urine cup to decrease the risk of contaminating the sample.
- Ⓟ Suprapubic aspiration is considered on children under the age of two with suspected sepsis or fever of unknown origin who are not toilet trained.
- Ⓟ Over the age of two, urethral catheterization is preferred over suprapubic urine aspiration for specimen collection.

- Ⓟ The majority of kidney stones will exit spontaneously without treatment.
- Ⓟ Rapid deceleration forces such as motor vehicle collisions or falling from a great height are common causes of renal trauma.
- Ⓟ Pediatric patients have a higher risk of bladder trauma than adults as the bladder is an abdominal organ and less protected in pediatric patients.
- Ⓟ Mild testicular trauma is treated with scrotal support, nonsteroidal anti-inflammatory medications, ice packs, and bed rest for 24—48 hours.
- Ⓟ Testicular torsion is more likely in males under 20 and epididymitis occurs more often in males over 20 years of age.
- Ⓟ Circumcised males are less likely to develop urinary tract infections than uncircumcised males.
- Ⓟ Yellow-brown urine often indicates bile in the blood from liver dysfunction.

Ⓟ Discomfort from renal colic is felt in the flank and abdomen on the same side as the kidney stone and may refer to the labia or scrotum.

Ⓟ 5—10% of pelvic fractures have concurrent bladder trauma.

Ⓟ Suprapubic urine aspiration should not be performed if the patient has voided within the past hour.

Ⓟ Patients who sustain a penile fracture often relate a popping sound at the time of the injury followed by discoloration and swelling of the penile shaft.

Ⓟ When a testicle twists on its spermatic cord, it becomes ischemic. This is termed a testicular torsion.

Ⓟ Indications of benign prostatic hypertrophy include urinary hesitation, urinary frequency, weak urinary stream, and nocturia.

Ⓟ Frequent urinary tract infections in school-aged children should raise the index of suspicion for congenital obstructive lesions, diabetes, or the possibility of sexual abuse.

- Ⓟ The bladder must be palpable or visualized on bladder scanner prior to attempting suprapubic catheterization.
- Ⓟ Inability of the liver to discard bilirubin in liver dysfunction may result in clay colored stools and brownish-colored urine.
- Ⓟ The urine test of a patient with renal colic may demonstrate hematuria, bacteremia, and proteinuria.
- Ⓟ In renal trauma, the left renal vein is injured more often than the right renal vein.
- Ⓟ A patient with bladder trauma may feel the need to void, but be unable to do so. Attempting to void may cause suprapubic pain in these patients.
- Ⓟ Ruptured testicles will require surgical repair.
- Ⓟ The pain of a testicular torsion usually has a rapid onset, whereas the pain of epididymitis has a more gradual onset.
- Ⓟ Prostatitis is most common in diabetic men, those with immunosuppressive conditions or patients undergoing renal dialysis.

- ⓟ Gonorrhea can contribute to the development of pelvic inflammatory disease.
- ⓟ Urethral or prostate infections are common causes of urinary tract infections in the adult male.
- ⓟ A minimum of 10 mL of urine is needed in the bladder for suprapubic urine aspiration.
- ⓟ A patient's serum creatinine must be less than 2mg/dL before intravenous contrast can be given.
- ⓟ Patients with fractures of the posterior lower ribs or spinous processes frequently have concomitant renal trauma.
- ⓟ Hypovolemia and hematuria are frequent findings with bladder injuries.
- ⓟ The majority of testicular torsions occur during adolescence.
- ⓟ 50% of testicular torsions occur during sleep, the other half are associated with heavy lifting, sporting activities, or testicular trauma.

- ⓟ Testicular inflammation is termed orchitis
- ⓟ Pyelonephritis in pregnancy is associated with premature delivery, preeclampsia, maternal anemia, and amnionitis.
- ⓟ During suprapubic urine aspiration, place a patient in the supine position with the knees flexed and the bottom of the heels as close to the perineum as possible.
- ⓟ Bowel trauma is frequently associated with trauma to the bladder.
- ⓟ Blunt trauma to the penis can cause a penile fracture.
- ⓟ A penile fracture occurs when the tunica albuginea is ruptured and blood extravasates into the penile shaft.
- ⓟ The usual cause of epididymitis in younger males is *Chlamydia trachomatis.*
- ⓟ Epididymitis in older males is most commonly caused by *E. Coli* secondary to underlying obstructive urinary disease.
- ⓟ Prostatitis is an inflammation of the prostate gland.

Ⓟ The most common causative agent of a urinary tract infection is *Escherichia coli.*

Ⓟ If a child does not void within 30 minutes of placing a urinary bag for a clean catch specimen, it should be removed, the area re-cleansed and a new bag placed to decrease contamination.

Ⓟ A full bladder at the time of injury increases the risk of bladder trauma.

Ⓟ Signs of testicular trauma include acute pain, nausea, vomiting, syncope and urinary retention.

Ⓟ Phimosis is a condition where the foreskin does not fully retract over the head of the penis.

Ⓟ Paraphimosis is a condition where the retracted foreskin of a penis causes a tight band around the head of the penis. This can lead to obstruction of urinary flow and ischemia to the head of the penis.

Ⓟ The neonatal age is the only point where males are more likely to develop a urinary tract infection then females.

- Ⓟ Colorless urine is associated with conditions such as diabetes insipidus, diuretic therapy, and diabetes mellitus in which the urine is dilute.
- Ⓟ Complete urinary obstructions caused by a kidney stone can result in pyelonephritis and post-renal failure.
- Ⓟ Rapid deceleration forces such as motor vehicle collisions or falling from a great height are common causes of renal trauma.
- Ⓟ Although less sensitive, renal sonography or magnetic resonance imaging (MRI) may be used to diagnose kidney stones in pregnant patients to decrease radiation exposure.
- Ⓟ Leaking of blood from bladder trauma can result in lower abdominal or perineal hematomas and abdominal distension.
- Ⓟ Elevating or manipulating the scrotum of a patient with testicular torsion will increase scrotal pain.
- Ⓟ Complications associated with untreated pyelonephritis include renal insufficiency, renal failure, perinephric abscess, and bacteremia.

- ℗ Chlamydia is a frequent cause of female infertility and nongonococcal urethritis in heterosexual males.
- ℗ Pyridium (phenazopyridine) causes the urine to turn an orange-red color.
- ℗ The majority of kidney stones are composed of calcium.
- ℗ Risk factors for calcium stones include high serum or urine calcium, alkaline urine, hyperparathyroidism and a family history of calcium stones.
- ℗ Clinical manifestations of renal trauma include hematuria as well as abdominal, flank and back tenderness or bruising.
- ℗ Elevation of the knees may relieve the pain associated with bladder trauma.
- ℗ Elevating the knees may increase intrathoracic or intracranial pressure and should be avoided in patients with suspected intracranial or intrathoracic trauma.
- ℗ The cremasteric reflex disappears on the side of a testicular torsion.

Ⓟ To elicit the cremasteric reflex, stimulate the inside of the male thigh. A positive reflex will result in elevation of the testicle on the side that is stimulated.

Ⓟ Pyruia is urine which contains pus.

Ⓟ Patients with calcium stones should be encouraged to avoid spinach, rhubarb, parsley, chocolate, cocoa, instant coffee, tea, and large amounts of milk.

Ⓟ Renal trauma may cause significant blood loss with signs of hypovolemia and an expanding flank mass.

Ⓟ If a concurrent urethral tear is not suspected with a fractured penis, a urinary catheter should be passed to prevent urinary obstruction from edema.

Ⓟ Epididymitis is usually described as a dull ache in the lower abdomen and scrotum.

Ⓟ Common causes of orchitis include mumps, under or untreated epididymitis.

Ⓟ Indications of a urinary tract infection in the infant include feeding difficulties, irritability, and hypothermia or hyperthermia.

Ⓟ When a urine sample is required from a menstruating woman, she should be catheterized to assure a non-contaminated sample.

Ⓟ Red or red-brown urine may be caused by excessive ingestion of beets, berries, fava beans, or red food coloring.

Ⓟ Chlamydia has been linked to preterm labor and postpartum endometriosis.

Ⓟ Patients with Herpes Simplex II should be taught to keep lesions clean and dry and avoid using lubricants and cream which can increase healing time.

Ⓟ Frequent urinary tract infections predispose patients to kidney stones composed of struvite.

Ⓟ Men are more likely to get calcium stones; women are more likely to get struvite stones.

- Ⓟ Male patients sustain urethral trauma more often then females because the urethra is more exposed in men.
- Ⓟ Children with urinary tract infections may demonstrate night enuresis or daytime incontinence.
- Ⓟ Pyrvinium pamoate (Povan) causes urine to turn red or reddish-brown.
- Ⓟ Risk factors for struvite kidney stones include alkaline urine, hyperparathyroidism, and frequent urinary tract infections.
- Ⓟ Acidic urine increases the risk of developing a uric acid stone.
- Ⓟ Acidification of urine with protein or fruit juice reduces the risk of developing a struvite kidney stone.
- Ⓟ Patients with suspected urethral tears or bladder ruptures should not be catheterized to prevent further damage.
- Ⓟ Suprapubic, instead of urethral catheters are usually placed when bladder ruptures or urethral tears are suspected or present.
- Ⓟ Gonorrhea and chlamydia are treated with antibiotics.

- ℗ The symptoms of Herpes Simplex II virus waxes and wanes, recurring an average of 3 – 4 times per year, typically following trauma to the genitalia or at times of high stress.
- ℗ Patients with gout have an increased risk of developing uric acid kidney stones.
- ℗ Elevation of the scrotum and wearing supportive garments may diminish the pain of epididymitis.
- ℗ To test for costovertebral angle tenderness, strike the costovertebral angle with the heel of the closed fist.
- ℗ Pseudomonas bacteria may cause urine to turn green.
- ℗ The most common site for blisters to appear with a Herpes Simplex II infection is the cervix and vulva on women, and the glans and prepuce on men.
- ℗ Jewish men carry a high risk of developing uric acid kidney stones.
- ℗ Acidic urine increases the risk of developing a uric acid stone.

Ⓟ In the absence of hemodynamic instability, renal trauma patients will usually be treated non-surgically.

Ⓟ The most common site of urethral trauma in women is the bladder neck and is often associated with obstetrical injuries, anterior vaginal lacerations, straddle injuries, and pelvic fractures.

Ⓟ The epididymis, which normally lies on the posterior surface of the testicle may be palpated on the anterior surface in patients with testicular torsion.

Ⓟ Benign prostatic hypertrophy increases the risk of urinary calculi, urinary tract infections, and ultimately, renal failure.

Ⓟ A kidney-ureter-bladder x-ray may reveal edema of a kidney in patients with pyelonephritis.

Ⓟ A diet high in purines increases the risk of developing a uric acid kidney stone.

Ⓟ Foods high in purine include organ meats like liver and kidney, sardines, herring, and goose.

Ⓟ The most common location of gonorrhea is the penis or vagina, although it can occur in the throat, the anus and in the eyes secondary to alternate sexual practices or childbirth.

Ⓟ In males, the anterior portion of the urethra is most often injured secondary to straddle injuries or a direct blow to the perineum.

Ⓟ In males, the posterior segment of the urethra is most often injured secondary to a direct blow to the perineum.

Ⓟ Women need to be encouraged to void frequently, completely and immediately after intercourse to avoid urinary tract infections.

Ⓟ Urine should be transported to the lab within one hour of collection or it begins to degrade.

Ⓟ If urine cannot be transported to the lab within one hour of collection, it should be refrigerated to prevent degradation and alteration of results.

Ⓟ Alkalinizing the urine reduces the risk of developing a uric acid kidney stone.

- ℗ Potassium citrate and Zyloprin (allopurinol) are used to alkalinize urine.
- ℗ Sexual activity, physical strain or exertion increases the pain of epididymitis.
- ℗ Discharge teaching for benign prostatic hypertrophy should include reducing alcohol and caffeine intake and avoiding fluid intake prior to bedtime to decrease nocturia.
- ℗ Resisting the urge to void may increase the risk of a urinary tract infection.
- ℗ When aspirating urine in a suprapubic urine aspiration, the needle is placed 1 – 2 cm above the symphysis pubis.
- ℗ Soaks, sitz baths, cool compresses, as well as wearing loose fitting clothing and cotton underwear may diminish the discomfort associated with the lesions of Herpes Simplex II.
- ℗ Aside from scrotal pain, symptoms of testicular torsion include nausea, vomiting, low grade fever, scrotal enlargement, redness, and pallor.

Ⓟ The pain of prostatitis is usually in the lower back or abdomen but may radiate to the penis, scrotum, perineum, or rectal area.

Ⓟ Chlamydia and gonorrhea often co-exist.

Ⓟ Patients with frequent urinary tract infections should be encouraged to wear cotton rather than synthetic underwear to reduce the risk of recurring infections.

Ⓟ There is no cure for Herpes Simplex II but antiviral medication can reduce the number of outbreaks,

Ⓟ Panty hose and other tight garments should not be worn by patients with frequent urinary tract infections or vulvovaginitis.

Ⓟ After the needle is withdrawn from a suprapubic urine aspiration, direct pressure should be applied for a minimum of three minutes.

Ⓟ Cystine kidney stones are rare and caused by a genetic defect which causes high serum cystine levels.

Ⓟ Hemodynamically unstable patients or those with evidence of renal pedicle injury will usually be treated surgically.

- Ⓟ Warm baths, topical anesthetics and analgesics may reduce pain and discomfort of Herpes Simplex II outbreaks.
- Ⓟ Bubble baths, perfumed soaps and douches may increase the risk of urinary tract infections and should be avoided by those at risk.
- Ⓟ Alkalinization of urine decreases the risk of cystine kidney stones.
- Ⓟ Uncircumcised male infants are often born with phimosis. This resolves with age.
- Ⓟ Because epididymitis is associated with infections, symptoms such as urinary frequency, urgency, dysuria, pyuria, fever, chills, and elevated white blood cell count are common.
- Ⓟ Common causes of prostatitis include recent urinary instrumentation, urinary tract infection, or benign prostatic hypertrophy.
- Ⓟ Indications of orchitis include hematuria, pain and swelling of the affected testicle and ejaculation of blood.
- Ⓟ Patients with urinary tract infections should be instructed to increase intake of fruit juices and protein to increase acidification of urine.

- Ⓟ Males who are suspected of having a sexually transmitted disease should be discouraged from giving a urine sample until a urethral swab is performed.
- Ⓟ Patients should not be discharged until they have voided following suprapubic urine aspiration.
- Ⓟ Typhus may cause urine to turn a dark brown or black color.
- Ⓟ Methylene blue can cause urine to turn dark brown or black.
- Ⓟ Patients discharged home with kidney stones need to be encouraged to increase fluid intake.
- Ⓟ Complete urethral tears may result in the inability to void with a distended, palpable bladder.
- Ⓟ Orchitis is treated with steroids, non-steroidal anti-inflammatory drugs, and elevation of the scrotum on an ice pack.
- Ⓟ Increased fluid intake may reduce the length and severity of a urinary tract infection.

- Ⓟ 100,000 colony-forming units of a single organism in a clean-catch specimen is considered diagnostic for a urinary tract infection.
- Ⓟ After suprapubic urine aspiration, voiding pink urine is normal, but frank hematuria is reason for concern.
- Ⓟ Patients with Herpes Simplex II should avoid intercourse when they have lesions. Intercourse is avoided until all genital lesions have crusted over. Barrier protection should be used between outbreaks.
- Ⓟ Hematuria may be microscopic or absent in as many as one-third of renal trauma patients.
- Ⓟ An aged urine specimen may appear cloudy.
- Ⓟ Narcotic or non-narcotic medications as well as anti-emetics, anti-inflammatory agents, antibiotics and antipyretics will be considered for kidney stones.
- Ⓟ Retrograde or computerized tomography cystography are used to diagnose urethral injuries.

Ⓟ Ice should be applied to a fractured penis and the patient prepared for surgical intervention.

Ⓟ Detorsion of a testicular torsion has the best results if it is performed within six hours. If a testicular torsion is not resolved within 12 hours, orchiectomy is likely.

Ⓟ Patients with epididymitis should maintain bed rest for 3 – 4 days and wear scrotal support when out of bed.

Ⓟ Gonorrhea and chlamydia in the female causes a thick yellow or white discharge 2-7 days after exposure followed by vaginal bleeding, vaginal itching, and dysuria.

Ⓟ Male patients with chlamydia infections may have a yellow-white thin discharge with burning on urination, urethral itching, and signs of epididymitis.

Ⓟ Ice should be applied to paraphimosis to facilitate manual retraction of the foreskin.

(P) Patients diagnosed with prostatitis should be encouraged to utilize sitz baths for pain relief, use stool softeners, and ensure adequate hydration.

(P) Patients being discharged home with kidney stones need to be encouraged to increase fluid intake and strain all urine until pain subsides or the stone passes.

(P) Women with Herpes Simplex II have an increased risk of cervical cancer and should be routinely monitored with pap smears.

Bibliography for genitourinary emergencies

Danis, D., Blansfield, J., & Gervasini, A. (2007). *Handbook of clinical trauma: the first hour* (4 ed.). St. Louis: Mosby Elsevier.

Honigman, B. K. (2005). *Emergency Medicine* (2 ed.). (mitchell, & e. L. Mitchell, Eds.) baltimore: Lippincott, Williams, Wilkins.

Hoyt, K. S., & Selfridge-Thomas, J. (Eds.). (2007). *Emergency Nursing Core Curriculum* (6 ed.). St. Louis: Saunders Elsevier.

Kunz Howard P, Steinmann, RA (Eds.) (2010). Sheehy's Emergency Nursing: Principles and Practice. 6th ed. St. Louis: Mosby.

Moses, S. (2010, March 22). *Clean catch urine collection*. Retrieved December 24, 2011, from Family practice notebook: http://www.fpnotebook.com/Urology/Lab/ClnCtchUrnClctn.htm

O'Toole, M. T. (Ed.). (2003). *Encyclopedia and dictionary of medicine, nursing and allied health* (7 ed.). St. Louis: Saunders Elsevier.

Proehl, J. (2009). *Emergency Nursing Procedures* (4 ed.). St. Louis: Saunders.

Gynecological

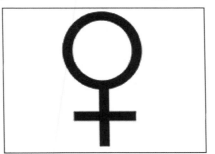

Emergencies

Ⓟ Bleeding secondary to a hormonal imbalance is termed dysfunctional uterine bleeding.

Ⓟ Changes in vaginal flora from pregnancy, recent antibiotic use, diabetes, HIV infection, high carbohydrate intake, poor hygiene practices and stress can cause vulvovaginitis.

Ⓟ Sitz baths can be used to relieve the discomfort of a Bartholin's cyst.

Ⓟ Pelvic inflammatory disease is an infection anywhere along the female reproductive tract including the endometrium, fallopian tubes, ovaries, pelvic peritoneum, or pelvic connective tissue.

Ⓟ Sexually assaulted patients should receive triage priority (after patients experiencing an acute life-threatening event) and should be placed in a safe secure room.

Ⓟ Dysfunctional uterine bleeding is often associated with anovulation and occurs more commonly at the beginning and end of the reproductive years.

Ⓟ Normal vaginal pH is 3.8.

Ⓟ The vaginal pH will elevate above 4.5 in patients with trichomonas vaginitis.

Ⓟ Two common causes of pelvic inflammatory disease are *N. gonorrhoeae* and *C. trachomatis.*

Ⓟ Ruptured blood filled ovarian cysts can lead to massive blood loss with resultant hypovolemic shock.

Ⓟ Causes of dysfunctional uterine bleeding may include low calorie diets, rapid weight change, obesity, thyroid or adrenal disorders, cirrhosis, and hypertension.

Ⓟ Bacterial vaginosis causes thin white discharge which adheres to vaginal walls.

Ⓟ Factors which increase the risk of pelvic inflammatory disease include sexually transmitted diseases, instrumentation, early sexual activity, and use of an intrauterine device.

ⓟ Medications linked to dysfunctional uterine bleeding include hormone replacement therapy, steroids, androgens, digitalis, and anticoagulants.

ⓟ Vaginal discharge associated with trichomonas vaginitis is watery, with a yellow, gray, or green color; and is often frothy or bubbly with a fishy odor that is notably worse after sexual intercourse.

ⓟ Patients with pelvic inflammatory disease may describe pelvic pain which worsens when they walk, defecate, urinate, perform Valsalva's maneuver, or have sexual intercourse.

ⓟ Follicular ovarian cysts usually cause pain in the first two weeks of the menstrual cycle and may rupture with strenuous exercise or sexual intercourse.

ⓟ Pain associated with the rupture of a cyst mid-cycle is termed Mittelschmerz.

ⓟ Rupture of a corpus luteum results in ovarian pain in the latter half of the cycle.

Ⓟ Breakthrough bleeding with contraceptive therapy is the most common cause of abnormal bleeding, often indicating poor compliance or inadequate daily doses.

Ⓟ Candida vulvovaginitis causes a white, curdy, "cottage-cheese like" vaginal discharge that adheres to vaginal walls.

Ⓟ Pelvic inflammatory disease secondary to *N. gonorrhoeae* will usually cause the greatest pelvic pain within 5 – 7 days of menstruation.

Ⓟ Sexual assault forensic exams will reveal the most useful information when performed within 72 hours of the assault, however evidence may be obtainable after that time frame.

Ⓟ Abnormal bleeding may occur secondary to therapeutic levels of anticoagulants.

Ⓟ The pain of pelvic inflammatory disease secondary to *C. trachomatis* is most often minimal and not related to menstruation.

Ⓟ Bacterial vaginosis is treated with antibiotics.

- ℗ Normal vaginal bleeding associated with menstruation is 25 – 60 mL per day for 4 to 5 days.
- ℗ Bacterial vaginosis is treated with antibiotics.
- ℗ Frequent causes of a Bartholin's cyst includes *E. Coli*, *G. vaginalis* or sexually transmitted diseases.
- ℗ Because walking can increase pelvic pain related to pelvic inflammatory disease (PID), patients may walk stooped forward, which is often referred to as the "PID shuffle."
- ℗ An average tampon holds 20 – 30 mL of blood when fully saturated.
- ℗ Trichomonas vaginitis is treated with Metronidazole (Flagyl) PO or clotrimazole vaginally.
- ℗ Patients who take Metronidazole (Flagyl) must be taught to abstain from alcohol while taking the medication and for 7 days after completing the medication to prevent an antabuse reaction.
- ℗ Excessive vaginal bleeding is defined as saturating more than one pad or tampon per hour for several consecutive hours.

- Ⓟ Common laboratory findings associated with pelvic inflammatory disease includes leukocytosis with a "shift to the left", elevated erythrocyte sedimentation rate and elevated C-reactive protein levels.
- Ⓟ Vaginal bleeding less than 21 days from the last episode of menstrual bleeding is termed dysfunctional uterine bleeding.
- Ⓟ Candida vulvovaginitis is treated with Gynazole (Butoconazole) cream intravaginally, Diflucan (Fluconazole) PO, or Clotrimazole (Lomotrin, Mycelex) intravaginally.
- Ⓟ The pain of an ovarian cyst usually results in a dull ache on the affected side and may result in prolonged menstruation.
- Ⓟ Vaginal bleeding associated with hormonal imbalances is usually painless; vaginal bleeding associated with endometriosis usually involves pain.

Bibliography for gynecological emergencies

Center for disease control and prevention. (2010, September 1). *Bacterial vaginosis*. Retrieved December 24, 2011, from Center for disease control and prevention: http://www.cdc.gov/STD/BV/STDFact-Bacterial-Vaginosis.htm#Treatment

Honigman, B. K. (2005). *Emergency Medicine* (2 ed.). (mitchell, & e. L. Mitchell, Eds.) baltimore: Lippincott, Williams, Wilkins.

Hoyt, K. S., & Selfridge-Thomas, J. (Eds.). (2007). *Emergency Nursing Core Curriculum* (6 ed.). St. Louis: Saunders Elsevier.

Kunz Howard P, Steinmann, RA (Eds.) (2010). Sheehy's Emergency Nursing: Principles and Practice. 6th ed. St. Louis: Mosby.

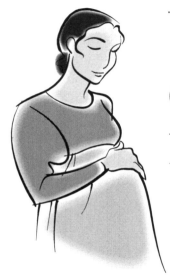

Obstetrical
Emergencies

ⓟ A spontaneous abortion is defined as a loss of pregnancy before the age of fetal viability.

ⓟ Complications of hyperemesis gravidarum include metabolic acidosis, ketonuria, hemoconcentration, gastrointestinal bleeding, and Wernicke's encephalopathy.

ⓟ All pregnant patients with vaginal bleeding should be assessed for hypovolemia.

ⓟ Hypertension after the twentieth week of pregnancy is termed gestational hypertension.

ⓟ Gestational hypertension with proteinuria is called pre-eclampsia.

ⓟ Hypovolemic shock should be treated aggressively in the pregnant patient since it can be detrimental to the unborn fetus.

ⓟ When preparing a mother for precipitous delivery she should be placed in the dorsal recumbent position with her knees bent or side-lying with the upper leg elevated.

Ⓟ When the umbilical cord precedes the infant out of the birth canal, it is termed a prolapsed cord.

Ⓟ Fetal heart tones can usually be assessed after the 10th to 12th week of pregnancy.

Ⓟ A Doppler is typically required to assess fetal heart tones between the 10th and 18th week of pregnancy.

Ⓟ Fetal heart tones can usually be auscultated with a stethoscope after the 18th to 20th week of pregnancy.

Ⓟ The majority of spontaneous abortions occur before the eighth week of pregnancy.

Ⓟ Gestational hypertension is more common in those under the age of 20 and over the age of 40.

Ⓟ Gestational hypertension is more common in primigravidas.

Ⓟ Risk factors for gestational hypertension includes chronic vascular disease, renal disease, diabetes, multiple fetuses, and hydatidiform mole.

- Ⓟ When a pregnant patient is involved in a traumatic incident, contractions may occur but are usually sporadic and will resolve without treatment.
- Ⓟ Fetal heart tones should be measured every time maternal vital signs are measured.
- Ⓟ To diminish perineal tearing, mothers should be encouraged to pant and gentle pressure should be placed against the fetal head during delivery to prevent an explosive delivery.
- Ⓟ Immediately after delivery, an infant should be warmed; its head placed in the sniffing position, and the airway cleared with a bulb syringe or suction catheter.
- Ⓟ A threatened abortion involves uterine cramping and bleeding with a closed cervical os.
- Ⓟ In normotensive women, an elevation of systolic blood pressure above 140 mm hg or a diastolic pressure above 90 mmHg is diagnostic of gestational hypertension.

Ⓟ In hypertensive women, an elevation of systolic blood pressure 30 mmHg and diastolic pressure 15 mmHg above their baseline is diagnostic for gestational hypertension.

Ⓟ The uterine fundus is normally at the symphysis pubis at 12 weeks gestation.

Ⓟ The uterine fundus is normally at the umbilicus at 20 weeks gestation.

Ⓟ A uterine fundus above the umbilicus generally indicates a viable pregnancy.

Ⓟ The uterine fundus is normally at the xiphoid process at 36 weeks.

Ⓟ Fetal heart tones are best auscultated with the mother in the supine position.

Ⓟ After delivery of the fetal head, check for the cord around the neck, and slip over the head between contractions if possible.

Ⓟ When suctioning a newborn, the mouth should be suctioned prior to the nose.

Ⓟ A patient with an inevitable abortion will have uterine cramping and vaginal bleeding. The cervical os will be open but the products of conception have not yet evacuated from the uterus.

Ⓟ A patient with an incomplete abortion will have vaginal bleeding and uterine cramping. The cervical os will be open, and tissue will be noted in the cervix.

Ⓟ Risk factors for placenta previa include multiparous women, advanced maternal age, pregnancies occurring in rapid succession, multiple gestation pregnancies, and smoking.

Ⓟ Aside from hypertension, symptoms of pregnancy induced hypertension include headache, epigastric or right upper quadrant pain, visual disturbances, and shortness of breath.

Ⓟ HELLP syndrome is a rare but potentially fatal complication of pregnancy.

Ⓟ HELLP is an acronym for **H**emolysis, **E**levated **L**iver enzymes, and **L**ow **P**latelet count.

Ⓟ The hematocrit tends to be lower during pregnancy secondary to increased fluid content which causes dilution of the serum.

Ⓟ Pregnant patients should be cared for in the lateral position unless it is contraindicated. In that case, the uterus should be manually displaced laterally to prevent venocaval compression syndrome.

Ⓟ Fetal heart tones are usually heard in the mother's right or left lower quadrant late in pregnancy.

Ⓟ During labor, fetal heart tones are heard best midway between the umbilicus and the symphysis pubis.

Ⓟ Fetal heart tones are usually heard above the umbilicus in breech presentations.

Ⓟ After birth, the Apgar score should be measured at one and five minutes.

Ⓟ The five components of the Apgar score are heart rate, respiratory effort, muscle tone, reflex irritability, and color.

Ⓟ An Apgar score of 7 – 10 is considered a good outcome, a score of 4 – 6 is considered a moderate outcome, and a score of 0 – 3 is considered a poor outcome.

Ⓟ The fallopian tube will usually rupture around the twelfth week of pregnancy in most ectopic pregnancies involving the fallopian tube.

Ⓟ Patients with pre-eclampsia may have proteinuria , elevated creatinine levels, and decreased urinary output.

Ⓟ Venocaval compression syndrome is marked by hypotension, nausea, vomiting, and tachycardia.

Ⓟ After birth, the umbilical cord should be clamped 4 – 5 centimeters from the infant's abdomen and 4 – 5 centimeters away from the mother. It should be cut between these clamps once it stops pulsating.

Ⓟ The maternal pulse and respiratory tend to be higher during pregnancy.

- ℗ Sterile equipment should be used to cut the umbilical cord after delivery. If sterile instruments are unavailable, the infant should be kept at or below the level of the mom until the cord is cut.
- ℗ ℗ Risk factors for abruptio placentae include maternal hypertension, advanced maternal age, trauma, illegal drug use, low socioeconomic status, and dietary deficiencies.
- ℗ If a newborn infant has poor color or a heart rate less than 100 beats per minute after applying positive-pressure ventilations for 90 seconds, intubation should be carried out.
- ℗ A prolapsed umbilical cord is an obstetrical emergency that results in fetal hypoxia.
- ℗ A patient with a complete abortion has light vaginal bleeding and mild uterine cramping, but all products of conception have evacuated the cervix.
- ℗ Premature labor is defined as labor before the 37th week of gestation.

Ⓟ Women who experience a missed abortion have retained products of conception after the cervical os recloses and are at risk of becoming septic.

Ⓟ Immediately after birth, if an infant's heart rate remains below 100 beats per minute, central cyanosis persists or respirations are gasping despite the delivery of oxygen, positive pressure ventilations should be started.

Ⓟ Magnesium sulfate may be used to reduce the risk of seizures in patients with pregnancy induced hypertension.

Ⓟ Dilatation and curettage is considered for incomplete, missed, and septic abortions.

Ⓟ Rh negative women who experience bleeding or trauma during pregnancy should receive Rh immune globulin (RhoGAM or Rhophylac).

Ⓟ Rupture of a tubal pregnancy is marked by a sudden sharp severe pain which may be accompanied by pain in one or both shoulders.

Ⓟ Abruptio placentae has been linked to increased risk of disseminated intravascular coagulation.

Ⓟ Severe symptoms associated with pregnancy induced hypertension may require a cesarean section.

Ⓟ High blood pressure associated with gestational hypertension may be treated with drugs such as hydralazine (Apresoloine), labetalol (Normodyne, Trandate), or nitrorusside (Nipride).

Ⓟ Normally, the blood pressure of a pregnant woman tends to be decreased during pregnancy when compared to her pre-pregnant state.

Ⓟ When assessing fetal heart tones, they should be counted for 30 to 60 seconds.

Ⓟ Oxytocin (Pitocin) or methylergonovine (Methergine) may be used to control hemorrhage associated with vaginal bleeding.

Ⓟ Symptoms of pregnancy induced hypertension may occur any time after the twentieth week of gestation and may commence as long as 72 hours post-delivery.

- Ⓟ Uterine rupture is a rare but deadly complication of trauma during pregnancy and more common in women who have had a cesarean section in the past.
- Ⓟ Positive-pressure ventilations on a newborn are delivered at 40-60 breaths per minute.
- Ⓟ When administering magnesium sulfate, monitor for symptoms of magnesium toxicity such as diminished deep tendon reflexes, hypotension, respiratory depression, and decreased urine output.
- Ⓟ Magnesium toxicity is treated with intravenous calcium gluconate.
- Ⓟ The white blood cell count tends to elevate as a normal variance in pregnancy.
- Ⓟ Severe abdominal pain that suddenly diminishes following trauma may be an indication of a uterine rupture.
- Ⓟ Aside from abdominal pain, signs and symptoms of uterine rupture include a tender uterus, a non- palpable uterine fundus, and fetal parts palpable outside the uterus.

Ⓟ A heart rate of less than 60 beats per minute after oxygen admini-stration or positive pressure ventilations on a new born infant re-quire initiation of cardiac compressions.

Ⓟ Women discharged home with a threatened abortion should be encouraged to maintain bedrest for 24 – 48 hours, or until vaginal bleeding stops.

Ⓟ Women of child-bearing age with lower abdominal pain or vaginal bleeding should be treated as ectopic pregnancies until proven otherwise.

Ⓟ Risk factors for hyperemesis gravidarum include primiparous women, multiple-gestation pregnancies, and women weighing more than 25% of their ideal body weight.

Ⓟ Placenta previa often involves bright red vaginal bleeding whereas abruptio placentae is often darker red vaginal bleeding.

Ⓟ When patients with pregnancy induced hypertension begin to seize, they are deemed to have eclampsia.

Ⓟ The seizures of eclampsia are treated with Lorazepam (Ativan), other medications to reduce blood pressure, and a cesarean section.

Ⓟ Uterine rupture requires emergency surgery to save the life of the fetus and the mother.

Ⓟ Fetal tachycardia is defined as a fetal heart rate above 160 beats per minute.

Ⓟ Fetal bradycardia is defined as a fetal heart rate below 120 beats per minute.

Ⓟ Chest compressions on a newborn infant should be at 90 per minute.

Ⓟ A mother who presents with a prolapsed cord should be positioned face down with her knees to her chest and her buttocks in the air.

Ⓟ Bleeding associated with abruptio placentae may accumulate in the uterus, resulting in an elevating fundal height. Dark red vaginal bleeding may or may not be present.

- Ⓟ Blood urea nitrogen and creatinine values are usually slightly lower as a normal variance during pregnancy.
- Ⓟ Clinical manifestations of HELLP syndrome include right upper quadrant pain, nausea and vomiting, and possible jaundice.
- Ⓟ The lab results associated with HELLP syndrome include elevated bilirubin levels, elevated liver enzymes, and a decreased platelet count.
- Ⓟ Breast-feeding after birth stimulates the release of oxytocin, facilitating uterine contractions and placental separation.
- Ⓟ When performing chest compressions on a newborn, use both thumbs on the lower third of the sternum, with fingers encircling and supporting the back.
- Ⓟ The chest of the newborn infant should be depressed approximately one third the anteroposterior diameter of the chest during chest compressions.

- Ⓟ Women with vaginal bleeding due to abortion should be encouraged to avoid sexual intercourse or douching, both of which can increase uterine cramping.
- Ⓟ A dextrose solution is often used to replace fluids lost with hyperemesis gravidarum to break the cycle of ketosis.
- Ⓟ Risk factors for ectopic pregnancy include history of pelvic inflammatory disease, salpingitis, fallopian tube surgery, tubal ligation, previous ectopic, or use of intrauterine device.
- Ⓟ Abruptio placentae can cause colicky abdominal pain, backache, uterine rigidity, and painful contractions.
- Ⓟ Carbon dioxide levels in arterial blood gases are usually lower during pregnancy.
- Ⓟ Delivery of the placenta generally occurs spontaneously 20 – 30 minutes after birth of the infant.
- Ⓟ One ventilation should be delivered for every three compressions when resuscitating a newborn.

ⓅⒶⒸ More than 750 milliliters of bright red blood, hypotension, tachycardia, and pale, cool, clammy skin are evidence of a post-partum bleed.

Ⓟ Sexual intercourse and douching can increase the risk of infection after abortion if the cervical os is still open.

Ⓟ Platelets and fibrinogen levels tend to climb as a normal variance during pregnancy.

Ⓟ In cases of the death of a pregnant mother, a cesarean section must be performed within 20 minutes of maternal death and preferably within 5 minutes for best fetal outcome.

Ⓟ Risk factors for premature labor include trauma, infections such as bacterial vaginosis and *Trichomoniasis,* shortened cervix, and history of previous premature births.

Ⓟ Fetal heart tone assessment during labor should occur between maternal contractions.

Ⓟ Epinephrine, naloxone, and glucose are the three most commonly delivered drugs during neonatal resuscitation.

Ⓟ If fluid resuscitation is required as part of neonatal resuscitation, it is given at a rate of 10 mL/kg.

Ⓟ After delivery of the plancenta, the fundus of the uterus should be palpated every five minutes. It should feel firm and the size of the grapefruit.

Ⓟ To massage a boggy fundus, the uterus is massaged by placing one hand at the symphysis pubis and the other at the uterine fundus and massaging until the uterus feels firm.

Ⓟ The use of sanitary napkins as opposed to tampons can reduce the risk of infection and sepsis after a spontaneous abortion.

Ⓟ Once rehydrated, patients with hyperemesis gravidarum should be encouraged to start on oral fluids as tolerated than advance to small frequent meals of easy-to-digest high energy foods.

℗ Mild cases of HELLP syndrome may be admitted for observation; however, severe cases usually require an emergent cesarean section.

℗ Placenta previa is usually painless whereas an abruptio placenta often involves abdominal pain.

℗ Encouraging breast feeding and administration of oxytocin are treatment considerations for a post-partum bleeding.

℗ Methotrexate (Folex) may be used to terminate fetal growth in an ectopic pregnancy if the risk of a fallopian tube rupture is low.

℗ Premature labor is marked by more than six contractions per hour or occurring at least every ten minutes.

℗ Placing a sterile gloved hand in the vaginal canal and pushing the fetal head off the cervix may decrease fetal hypoxia with a prolapsed cord.

℗ A Kleihauer-Betke test is drawn to determine if there has been mixing of maternal and fetal blood.

Ⓟ The cervical os is open in an inevitable and incomplete abortion, but is closed in a threatened abortion.

Ⓟ The maternal pulse should be palpated simultaneously with auscultation for fetal heart tones to assure the maternal heart beat is not being counted.

Ⓟ Tubal pregnancies often start as a vague discomfort which progress to sharp colicky pain.

Bibliography for obstetrical emergencies

Hammond, BB. Gerber-Zimmerman, P. (Ed.). (2013). *Sheehy's manual of emergency care* (7 ed.). St. Louis: Mosby.

Honigman, B. K. (2005). *Emergency Medicine* (2 ed.). (mitchell, & e. L. Mitchell, Eds.) Baltimore: Lippincott, Williams, Wilkins.

Hoyt, K. S., & Selfridge-Thomas, J. (Eds.). (2007). *Emergency Nursing Core Curriculum* (6 ed.). St. Louis: Saunders Elsevier.

Kunz Howard P, Steinmann, RA (Eds.) (2010). Sheehy's Emergency Nursing: Principles and Practice. 6th ed. St. Louis: Mosby.

National institutes of health. (2010, August 2). *Preterm labor and birth*. Retrieved December 24 2011, from National Institute of child health and human development: http://www.nichd.nih.gov/health/topics/ Preterm_Labor_and_Birth.cfm

O'Toole, M. T. (Ed.). (2003). *Encyclopedia and dictionary of medicine, nursing and allied health* (7 ed.). St. Louis: Saunders Elsevier.

Probst, B. D. (2012). Emergency childbirth. In J. R. Roberts, & J. R. Hedges (Eds.), *Clinical procedures in emergency medicine* (5 ed., pp. 1042—1062). Philadelphia: Saunders.

Proehl, J. (2009). *Emergency Nursing Procedures* (4 ed.). St. Louis: Saunders

RESPIRATORY

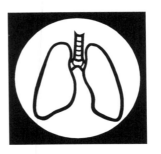

EMERGENCIES

Ⓟ Positive pressure ventilation prior to intubation increases the risk of aspiration.

Ⓟ Hypoxemia may result from prolonged suctioning, therefore suctioning should be limited to 10 seconds per approach.

Ⓟ When administering oxygen via nasal cannula, FiO_2 increases by 3 – 4% per liter increase in flow rate.

Ⓟ Oxygen via nasal cannula at one liter flow delivers approximately 24% oxygen, at two liters: 28%, at three liters: 32% and so on.

Ⓟ Continuous positive airway pressure (CPAP) is an oxygen delivery method which forces gases into the lungs equally through inhalation and exhalation.

Ⓟ Wheezes on auscultation are caused by narrowing of the lower, smaller airways.

Ⓟ Bilevel positive airway pressure (BiPAP) is an oxygen delivery method which forces higher pressures of gas during inhalation and less pressures during exhalation.

- Ⓟ Ideally, a bag-mask device should be attached to an oxygen source set at 10 to 15 liters/minute. If an oxygen source is unavailable, bag-mask ventilation can be used on room air.
- Ⓟ To estimate the diameter of an endotracheal tube on a patient, look at the diameter of the fifth (or pinky) finger. The two diameters should be the same.
- Ⓟ Laryngeal mask airways are more effective than a bag-mask device and may be considered as a temporary airway maintenance measure until endotracheal intubation can be performed.
- Ⓟ A needle cricothyrotomy is an emergent procedure that involves placing a hole in the exterior of the neck through the cricothyroid membrane into the trachea.
- Ⓟ Eupnea is used to describe respirations of normal rate and depth.
- Ⓟ An Allen's test is performed to determine patency of the ulnar artery.
- Ⓟ An asthma attack which does not respond to standard treatment is termed status asthmaticus.

Ⓟ When assisting with a thoracentesis, assist the patient to assume a seated position, leaning forward on a bedside table with the arms crossed.

Ⓟ Peak expiratory flow rate (PEFR) is an objective measurement of air flow. This test measures how fast the maximum amount of air can be expired during a forced expiration.

Ⓟ Chronic bronchitis causes production of excess pulmonary secretions and inability to clear those secretions coupled with diminished pulmonary defense mechanisms.

Ⓟ Acute bronchitis is an inflammation of the bronchi and/or trachea.

Ⓟ There are four types of pulmonary edema: cardiogenic, acute respiratory distress syndrome, neurogenic pulmonary edema and high altitude pulmonary edema.

Ⓟ For children over the age of two, add 16 to the child's age in years and divide that number by four to obtain the appropriate endotracheal tube size. (16+age in years/4)

- ℗ Blood clots from the right side of the heart, the pelvis or from a deep vein thrombosis in the legs are the most common causative agents of a pulmonary embolism.
- ℗ Large round or expandable objects tend to cause complete airway obstructions, irregularly shaped objects are more likely to cause partial airway obstructions.
- ℗ The spleen lies under ribs 10 through 12 on the left side. Rib fractures in this area are associated with splenic injury 20% of the time.
- ℗ Extravasation of blood into the lung parenchyma following chest trauma is known as a pulmonary contusion; frequently associated with rib fractures and flail chest segments.
- ℗ When administering oxygen via simple mask, the flow rate should be at least 5 – 6 liters per minute to minimize re-breathing of carbon dioxide.
- ℗ Fluid in the pleural space is called a pleural effusion.

Ⓟ Suctioning can increase intracranial pressure and should be used cautiously in patients with head injuries.

Ⓟ Paralytics and lidocaine administered prior to suctioning can minimize increases in intracranial pressure associated with suctioning the head injured patient.

Ⓟ In order for a laryngeal mask airway to be inserted, the patient must be unresponsive with absent glossopharyngeal and laryngeal reflexes.

Ⓟ Accumulation of more than 1000 milliliters of blood in a chest drainage system initially may indicate arterial bleeding and the need for surgery, therefore the physician should be notified.

Ⓟ A thoracentesis may be performed instead of a chest tube insertion for small accumulations of air or fluid in the pleural space.

Ⓟ When measuring peak expiratory flow rate, have the patient sit upright with the legs dangling to maximize diaphragmatic excursion.

Ⓟ A patient with status asthmaticus will have diminishing wheezes on auscultation until the chest becomes silent.

- Ⓟ Causes of acute bronchitis include viruses associated with upper respiratory tract infections and irritation of the upper airways from pollen, smoking or inhaling irritating substances.
- Ⓟ Decreased cardiac output, especially from the left ventricle, can cause fluid to back up into the lungs contributing to cardiogenic pulmonary edema.
- Ⓟ Fat emboli may be mobilized 24 to 48 hours after long bone fracture such as a fracture of the femur, humerus or pelvis.
- Ⓟ Metallic and caustic foreign objects in the airway can erode it resulting in ulceration and perforation of tissue if the object is not immediately removed.
- Ⓟ Pulmonary contusions tend to worsen with time. The patient may be mildly symptomatic on arrival to the ED with progression of symptoms throughout the ED stay or after admission.
- Ⓟ The liver lies under ribs 8 through 12 on the right side. Rib fractures in this area are associated with liver injury 10% of the time.

Ⓟ The prevention of complete expulsion of air on exhalation (leaving the alveoli partially inflated at the end of exhalation) is referred to as positive end expiratory pressure (PEEP).

Ⓟ The mask of an adequately sized bag-mask device should be large enough to seal around the mouth and nose without covering the eyes.

Ⓟ The usual size of endotracheal tube required for most adult men is 7.5 to 9 millimeters. The usual size of endotracheal tube required for most adult women is 7 to 8 millimeters.

Ⓟ Tachypnea is used to describe respirations of rapid rate regardless of depth (depth is variable).

Ⓟ Rhonchi are a snoring, low-pitched sound associated with narrowing of the large upper airways.

Ⓟ Pediatric sized laryngeal mask airways are available.

Ⓟ If a high pressure alarm sounds on the ventilator, check to make sure all the tubing between the ventilator and the patient is patent and not kinked.

- Ⓟ If a high pressure alarm sounds on the ventilator, make sure that the patient is not biting on the endotracheal tube, partially or completely occluding it.
- Ⓟ If a high pressure alarm sounds on the ventilator, check to see that the patient is not waking up and resisting or "bucking" the ventilator.
- Ⓟ Possible causes of high pressure alarms on a ventilator include development of a pneumothorax, bronchospasm or significant increases of fluid in the lungs.
- Ⓟ The pH of arterial blood is normally between 7.35 and 7.45. A pH above 7.45 is considered alkaline, a pH below 7.35 is considered acidotic.
- Ⓟ Blood in the pleural space is called a hemothorax.
- Ⓟ Lidocaine may be given prior to intubation as an anti-arrhythmic, as well as to blunt the gag and cough reflex and diminish elevations in intracranial pressure.

Ⓟ Hyperventilation is used to describe respirations of increased depth regardless of rate (rate is variable).

Ⓟ Atropine may be given prior to intubation, especially in children, to decrease the risk of bradycardia associated with vagal stimulation.

Ⓟ Accumulation of more than 200 milliliters of blood per hour for 3 to 4 hours in a chest drainage system may indicate arterial bleeding in the pleural space and the need for surgery.

Ⓟ Instruct the patient not to cough during a thoracentesis to prevent damage to the lung.

Ⓟ Chronic obstructive pulmonary disease involves three disease entities: asthma (reactive airway disease), chronic bronchitis (inflammatory disease) and emphysema (airway collapse).

Ⓟ To test peak expiratory flow rate, have the patient inhale fully and while holding the breath, place the mouth firmly about the mouthpiece, sealing the circumference. Once a seal is made, the patient should exhale as forcefully as possible.

- Ⓟ The onset of chronic bronchitis is typically between the ages of 40 and 50 years old.
- Ⓟ Aspiration pneumonitis is chemical damage to the tracheobronchial tree secondary to the aspiration of gastric contents.
- Ⓟ Common causes of cardiogenic pulmonary edema include heart failure, myocardial infarction, severe anemia, hyperthyroidism, hypertension, cardiomyopathies and myocarditis.
- Ⓟ An amniotic fluid bolus may occur within minutes after delivery of an infant.
- Ⓟ Partial obstructions of the larynx cause hoarseness and aphonia.
- Ⓟ Partial obstructions of the trachea cause wheezing similar to asthma. .
- Ⓟ Complete obstructions of the larynx and trachea cause complete airway obstruction with lack of coughing, airway sounds or air movement.
- Ⓟ Bronchiolitis is an inflammation of the small lower airways.

ⓟ Obstructions of the bronchi cause a cough, unilateral wheezing and a unilateral decrease in breath sounds on auscultation.

ⓟ Symptoms of a pulmonary contusion include dyspnea, hemoptysis, hypoxia, and obvious trauma to the external chest wall, with local or diffuse crackles as the condition progresses.

ⓟ The first and second ribs are strong bones, and are protected under the clavicle. Fractures to these ribs are often associated with significant underlying cardiothoracic trauma.

ⓟ Fractures of the first and second ribs are also associated with injury to the subclavian artery or vein and can result in significant hypovolemia.

ⓟ When using a bag-mask device, the proper size bag for infants and children is 450 – 500 milliliters and for adults, it is 1600 milliliters.

ⓟ Oxygen via simple mask may cause drying of the eyes.

ⓟ If nasotracheal intubation is being considered, the tube should be 0.5 to 1 millimeter smaller than the tube used for oral intubation.

- Ⓟ Conditions which tend to benefit from CPAP and BiPAP therapy include exacerbation of chronic obstructive pulmonary disease (COPD), acute respiratory failure, and acute cardiogenic pulmonary edema.
- Ⓟ After placing a laryngeal mask airway, check placement by assessing breath sounds, then inflate the cuff. The patient may then be ventilated using a bag-mask device.
- Ⓟ The depth of respirations in hyperventilation exceeds the metabolic demands of the body, therefore the patient will have high oxygen and low carbon dioxide content.
- Ⓟ Normally, carbon dioxide in the blood is between 35 and 45 mm Hg. Excess carbon dioxide contributes to respiratory acidosis, insufficient carbon dioxide contributes to respiratory alkalosis.
- Ⓟ Bicarbonate in the blood is normally between 22 and 26 mEq/L. Excess bicarbonate is associated with metabolic alkalosis, insufficient bicarbonate is associated with metabolic acidosis.

Ⓟ A simple pneumothorax is where air escapes into the pleural space by a hole from within the lungs or upper airway structures.

Ⓟ Common causes of a simple pneumothorax include trauma, baro-trauma, emphysema or spontaneously in tall, slender males who smoke.

Ⓟ A spontaneous pneumothorax is most common in young men between the ages of 20 and 40 with the highest incidence in the early 20s.

Ⓟ A hydrothorax is a collection of serous fluid in the pleural space associated with conditions such as left ventricular failure, liver failure and pulmonary embolism.

Ⓟ Patients with large volumes of blood in the pleural space may require fluid resuscitation prior to insertion of a chest tube.

Ⓟ In 50% of patients with asthma, the onset is before the age of ten. In some people, the disease will resolve with age, but 30% of those diagnosed with asthma in childhood will go on to have it as adults.

- ℗ Bronchodilators re-open constricted airways during asthma exacerbation.
- ℗ Common bronchodilators include epineneprhine (Adrenalin), racemic epinephrine (Micronefrin, Asthma Nefrin), terbutaline (Brethaire, Brethine), albuterol (Proventil, Ventolin), isoetherine (Bronkosol, Bronkometer), and salmeterol zinaoate (Serevent).
- ℗ Spacers increase vaporization of particles from a metered dose inhaler. This will increase lung penetration and decrease loss of drug into the air or mouth.
- ℗ It takes less coordination to use a spacer then a metered dose inhaler and may be an alternative to people who struggle with metered dose inhalers.
- ℗ Cor pulmonale is right-sided heart failure associated with respiratory problems.
- ℗ Dry powder inhalers are another alternative for people who cannot use a metered dose inhaler. This method is capable of high inspiratory volumes.

Ⓟ Symptoms of chronic bronchitis include a productive cough, hypoxemia, hypercarbia, chronic cyanosis, polycythemia, and right sided heart failure.

Ⓟ 90% of the time, bronchiolitis is caused by the highly contagious respiratory synctytial virus (RSV).

Ⓟ Aspiration pneumonia occurs when pnuemonitis progresses to pneumonia or may be caused by inhalation of small amounts of oropharyngeal contents (leading to pulmonary infections).

Ⓟ Acute respiratory distress syndrome is a non-cardiogenic pulmonary edema. Many times the patient's heart is perfectly healthy.

Ⓟ Acute respiratory distress syndrome is a caused by a leakage of fluids into the lungs secondary to initiation of the inflammatory system.

Ⓟ Air emboli are associated with inadvertent injection of air into an intravenous line or from rapid expansion of air in the alveoli when a diver surfaces too rapidly.

(P) Women have higher rates of pulmonary emboli because of the use of oral contraceptives and because of increased coagulation associated with pregnancy.

(P) When using a simple face mask, a flow of 5 – 6 liters of oxygen results in an FiO_2 of approximately 40%, at 6 – 7 liters, the FiO_2 goes up to 50%, and at 7 – 8 liters: 60%.

(P) A properly fitted mask with a seal is essential to use of BiPAP and CPAP. Air leaks around the mask will decrease the effectiveness of therapy.

(P) Defasciculating agents such as Vancuronium (Norcuron) or Pancuronium (Pavulon) may be given prior to intubation to decrease muscle fasciculations.

(P) Muscle fasciculations are commonly associated with the administration of succinycholine.

(P) Laryngeal mask airways and combitubes may be placed without the use of a laryngoscope.

- ℗ A jet ventilator device is used to ventilate a needle cricothyrotomy. The device forces air into the cricothyrotomy with pressures between 40 and 50 pounds per square inch (PSI).
- ℗ A patient must be able to hold their breath in order to use a metered dose inhaler.
- ℗ Hyperpnea is used to describe respirations in which both rate and depth are increased in response to the metabolic demands of the body, therefore oxygen and carbon dioxide levels are normal.
- ℗ Nasal flaring is an early indicator of respiratory distress in pediatric patients but a later indicator in adults.
- ℗ A pleural friction rub is a grating sound heard with inspiration and expiration associated with inflammation of the pleural surfaces.
- ℗ When performing rapid sequence intubation, an induction agent is given to cause loss of consciousness followed by a neuromuscular blocking agent.

℗ Conditions which impede respiratory drive (over-sedation or respiratory arrest) or airway obstruction (foreign objects or asthma) may contribute to respiratory acidosis.

℗ Neuromuscular disorders which impede the respiratory drive (Guillain-Barré or myasthenia gravis) can cause respiratory acidosis.

℗ Conditions that impair chest wall expansion such as chest injuries or abdominal distension can lead to respiratory acidosis.

℗ Pus in the pleural space is known as a pyothorax.

℗ To perform an Allen's test, have the patient elevate the hand above the level of the heart and open and close the fist several times. Then occlude the ulnar and radial arteries until the hand blanches. Next, release pressure on the ulnar artery while maintaining pressure on the radial artery.

℗ When releasing pressure on the ulnar artery as part of the Allen's test, the hand should flush in less than 7 seconds indicating a patent ulnar artery.

- Ⓟ When releasing pressure on the ulnar artery as part of the Allen's test, if it takes 8 to 14 seconds for the hand to flush, it is considered an equivocal finding.
- Ⓟ When releasing pressure on the ulnar artery as part of the Allen's test, if it takes longer than 14 seconds for the hand to flush, it is an abnormal finding and the radial artery should not be used for drawing arterial blood gases.
- Ⓟ Gentle bubbling on inspiration is a normal finding in the water seal chamber when a patient has a pnuemothorax.
- Ⓟ Once the needle is removed following a thoracentesis, a sterile dressing is applied to the area and a chest x-ray is performed.
- Ⓟ Bronchodilators have beta-two effects leading to bronchodilation and increased respiratory effects, but also have varying beta-one effects.
- Ⓟ Nebulizers are preferred for a patient who is unable or too sick to cooperate with metered dose inhalers and spacers.

Ⓟ Asthma is the most common chronic childhood illness.

Ⓟ In status asthmaticus, peak expiratory flow rate (PEFR) drops to less than 100L/minute in adults . (Inability to participate in PEFR measurement is a poor indicator of outcome).

Ⓟ Bronchiolitis is most common in children under one year of age and if it affects adults, it is usually mild.

Ⓟ Neurogenic pulmonary edema is rare and occurs within hours of a severe neurological insult.

Ⓟ Sudden onset of shortness of breath that cannot be explained for any other reason should always raise the index of suspicion for a pulmonary embolism.

Ⓟ The chest radiograph with a pulmonary contusion may appear normal during the initial presentation, but appear cloudy with time.

Ⓟ When delivering oxygen via non-rebreather, insufficient oxygen flow may lead to re-breathing of CO_2, therefore the oxygen level should be high enough that the reservoir bag never collapses.

Ⓟ When ventilating with a bag-mask device, a tidal volume of 6 to 7 mL/kg should be used if the device is hooked up to oxygen, 10 mL/kg is utilized if the device is being used on room air.

Ⓟ The proper depth of a tracheal tube is approximately 21 centimeters from the incisors for women and 23 centimeters from the incisors for men.

Ⓟ If using jet insufflation to ventilate a needle cricothyrotomy site, inhalation should be allowed to occur over one second, exhalation over 4 seconds.

Ⓟ Kussmaul's respirations are rapid and deep breathing without pauses. The patient appears to be air hungry or gasping to breathe.

Ⓟ Kussmaul's respirations are associated with states of acidosis.

Ⓟ Respiratory acidosis may cause central nervous system depression with symptoms such as decreased mentation, restlessness, somnolence, and lethargy.

- Ⓟ The percussion note of resonance heard over lung tissue indicates that tissue is free from disease.
- Ⓟ Respiratory acidosis may cause neuromuscular symptoms such as fatigue, muscle weakness, tremors, decreased reflexes and incoordination.
- Ⓟ Respiratory acidosis may cause vasodilation resulting in headaches and hypotension.
- Ⓟ The water seal in a chest drainage system should elevate slightly when a patient inhales.
- Ⓟ To obtain a radial blood gas sample, a small rolled towel or washcloth should be placed under the wrist so it is dorsiflexed 30 degrees.
- Ⓟ Cover an open pneumothorax with an occlusive dressing. Ideally, the dressing is placed at the height of inspiration.
- Ⓟ Epinephrine (Adrenalin) is a strong beta-two stimulant with rapid bronchodilation but significant beta-one stimulation.

Ⓟ When applying an occlusive dressing over an open pneumothorax, only tape the dressing on three sides to allow the escape of air in the un-taped side and prevent a tension pneumothorax.

Ⓟ Asthma is more prevalent among lower income, inner city black children, children with low birth weight, children of young mothers and those with allergies that lead to skin rashes.

Ⓟ Nebulizers deliver drugs to the lower airways better than other methods such as metered dose inhalers or spacers.

Ⓟ Chronic bronchitis is frequently associated with long-term smoking.

Ⓟ Pneumonia is an infection of the lung parenchyma resulting from tissue invasion by inhaled, aspirated or bloodborne pathogens.

Ⓟ Within 2 to 4 days after rapid ascent to an altitude above 8000 feet (2440 meters), patients may develop pulmonary edema.

Ⓟ Patients who live above 8000 feet (2440 meters) are unlikely to develop high altitude pulmonary edema unless they descend below that altitude for a few weeks then return home.

- Ⓟ Tachypnea and tachycardia are the most common findings associated with a pulmonary embolism.
- Ⓟ The ribs of pediatric patients are soft and pliable, therefore, rib fractures are less common in this age group.
- Ⓟ Signs of tracheobronchial injury include pain, some degree of dyspnea on arrival, hoarseness, hemoptysis and stridor.
- Ⓟ Of all oxygen delivery methods, a non-rebreather mask offers the highest oxygen delivery concentration.
- Ⓟ Diaphragmatic tears occur on the left side more than the right.
- Ⓟ Air leaks associated with BiPAP and CPAP can be remedied by choosing a smaller mask.
- Ⓟ Suctioning can stimulate the vagal response, leading to bradycardia and hypotension. This is especially true in the pediatric population.
- Ⓟ Oxygen flow must exceed 10 liters per minute when utilizing a non-rebreather mask.

- Ⓟ Nasal masks associated with BiPAP and CPAP cover the nose, but not the mouth. The patient must keep their mouth shut in order for this treatment to be effective.
- Ⓟ To estimate the appropriate depth of an endotracheal tube on pediatric patients, multiple the diameter of the tube by three.
- Ⓟ In patients with spontaneous respirations or an intact gag reflex, nasotracheal, rather than oral intubation may be considered.
- Ⓟ When using jet insufflations to ventilate a needle cricothyrotomy, the oxygen source should be set to 15 liters per minute.
- Ⓟ Dyspnea is a subjective sensation of difficult or labored breathing.
- Ⓟ To obtain an arterial blood gas, the needle should be inserted at the point of maximal impulse and should not be inserted if a pulse cannot be palpated.
- Ⓟ Hyperventilation and increased respiratory rates (from causes such as anxiety, exercise, high tidal volumes or respiratory rates on the ventilator) may cause respiratory alkalosis.

Ⓟ Acute hypoxemia, tissue acidosis (from causes such as sepsis, lactic academia) and hypermetabolic states (fever, pain, agitation, thyrotoxicosis) can result in respiratory alkalosis.

Ⓟ Drugs which increase the respiratory rate (aspirin, theophyllines, catecholamines, progesterone, acute alcohol intoxication) may all contribute to respiratory alkalosis.

Ⓟ Continuous bubbling in the suction control chamber of a chest drainage system indicates a patent suction system.

Ⓟ The percussion note of hyporesonance is a flat dull sound heard over solid tissue. When heard over lung tissue, suspect pleural effusion or pneumonia.

Ⓟ Patients should be seated upright at 40 to 90 degrees for nebulizer treatments.

Ⓟ Peak expiratory flow rates should be measured three times, choosing the best reading of the three. Expected values vary depending on a patient's sex, age and height.

Ⓟ A reading of 40 to 69% of what is expected for the patient is considered a moderate exacerbation of asthma, a reading of less than 40% is considered a severe exacerbation.

Ⓟ Emphysema is marked by loss of elasticity in the lung tissue, causing the trapping of air in the lungs, making them overdistended.

Ⓟ Causes of pneumonia include viruses (most common), bacteria (more serious infection then viral), fungi, rickettsiaes, parasites and mycoplasms.

Ⓟ Acute bronchitis starts with a dry, hacky nonproductive cough most troublesome at night; triggered by deep breathing, talking, and laughing. The cough becomes productive with time.

Ⓟ Any condition which reduces a patient's gag reflex or ability to protect their own airway puts them at risk for either aspiration pneumonitis or pneumonia.

Ⓟ Aside from shortness of breath, other symptoms of a pulmonary embolism include cough, hemoptysis, diaphoresis, syncope, fever and crackles on auscultation.

- Ⓟ Elderly patients with rib fractures are more likely to be admitted then younger people with rib fractures as they are more likely to require pulmonary care.
- Ⓟ A CT scan is more sensitive to diagnose a pulmonary contusion immediately after the injury then a chest radiograph.
- Ⓟ The usual place for air leaks when using nasal masks in CPAP and BiPAP therapy is the bridge of the nose.
- Ⓟ Nasotracheal intubation is not performed on the apneic patient or patients with suspected facial, nasal or basilar skull fractures.
- Ⓟ After placement of a combitube, the blue ventilation tube should be ventilated first as this tube is most often in the trachea.
- Ⓟ If indications of adequate ventilation (chest rise and fall, adequate bilateral breath sounds, etc.) do not occur when ventilating the blue tube of a combitube, ventilate the white tube.
- Ⓟ When using a combitube, the tube which does not result in chest ventilation can be used as a passage for a gastric tube.

Ⓟ If the cause of a high pressure alarm on a ventilator cannot be easily determined, consider suctioning the patient.

Ⓟ Bradypnea is used to describe slow respirations regardless of depth (depth is variable).

Ⓟ The percussion note of hyperresonance is a high pitched tympanic note associated with hyperinflation diseases of the lung such as emphysema or a pneumothorax.

Ⓟ To obtain an arterial blood gas, the needle is inserted at a 30 to 45 degree angle.

Ⓟ An iatrogenic simple pneumothorax is a pneumothorax that is caused by a medical procedure.

Ⓟ Common causes of an iatrogenic simple pneumothorax include central line insertions, mechanical ventilation with high peak end expiratory pressures and intubation of the patient in status asthmaticus.

Ⓟ Orthopnea is a sensation of dyspnea when lying down.

Ⓟ Lymphatic fluid may spill from the thoracic duct into the pleural space causing a chylothorax. This may occur with chest trauma or lymphomas.

Ⓟ Water-seal chest drainage devices must be kept upright otherwise, the system is no longer patent and air may re-enter into the pleural space, re-expanding a pneumothorax.

Ⓟ Racemic epinephrine (Micronefrin, Asthma Nefrin) has strong beta-two stimulation with ½ the beta-one effects found in epinephrine (Adrenalin).

Ⓟ A patient in status asthmaticus will be unable to speak or lie flat and oxygen saturations will often be below 90% despite supplemental oxygen.

Ⓟ Patients with chronic bronchitis and emphysema have diminished pulmonary defense mechanisms and are at increased risk of developing lung infections.

Ⓟ Suctioning can stimulate the gag reflex, increasing the risk of vomiting and aspiration.

Ⓟ Aside from a cough, bronchitis can cause chest pain and is usually accompanied by signs of upper respiratory tract infections. (sore throat, stuffy nose, cough, etc.).

Ⓟ Examples of conditions which increase this risk of aspiration pneumonitis or pneumonia include cerebrovascular accident, head trauma, alcohol intoxication, or drug overdose.

Ⓟ Patients with pulmonary emboli may experience the sudden onset of pleuritic chest pain that increases during inspiration.

Ⓟ Patients with underlying pulmonary disease, such as chronic obstructive pulmonary disease, carry a higher risk of pulmonary complications after rib fractures.

Ⓟ Air entrapment masks (Venturi masks) allow precise control of FiO_2 and are particularly useful for chronic obstructive pulmonary disease patients where tight control of oxygen levels is important.

Ⓟ Gurgling sounds over the epigastrium coupled with lack of chest movement is a strong indicator of esophageal endotracheal tube placement.

- ℗ Fast and deep breathing punctuated by periods of apnea is referred to as Biot's respirations.
- ℗ Biot's respirations are related to damage to the medulla oblongata from strokes or trauma. These respirations may also be seen in meningitis.
- ℗ Intercostal muscle retractions are early indicators of respiratory distress in children but a later indicator in adults.
- ℗ Cricoid pressure (Sellick's maneuver) is used to prevent aspiration of gastric contents and improve visualization of the vocal cords during intubation.
- ℗ Cricoid pressure (Sellick's maneuver) is defined as the application of backward pressure on the cricoid cartilage to occlude the esophagus.
- ℗ Do not clamp a chest tube unless it is absolutely necessary, as clamping can increase intrapleural pressure and contribute to a tension pneumothorax.

Ⓟ Clamping a chest tube may be necessary to change a chest drainage device or to check for air leaks.

Ⓟ Asthma triggers include allergen inhalation (animal danders, house dust mites, pollens and molds), upper respiratory viral infections, food additives, menses and cold, dry air.

Ⓟ Additional asthma triggers include air pollutants (exhaust fumes, perfumes, oxidants, sulfur dioxides, cigarette smoke, aerosol sprays), sulfites (bisulfites and metabisulfites) and tartrazine.

Ⓟ Additional asthma triggers include exercise (asthma may flare up 10 – 20 minutes after exercise.) gastroesophageal reflux disease and emotional stress.

Ⓟ Drugs known to exacerbate asthma include aspirin, non-steroidal anti-inflammatory drugs and beta-adrenergic blockers.

Ⓟ Terbutaline (Brethaire, Brethine) lasts four to six hours and is beta-two specific with less beta-one effects than many other bronchodilators.

Ⓟ If the heart rate increases more than 20 beats per minute during a nebulized treatment, stop the treatment. In pregnant patients, don't forget to assess fetal heart rate when administering nebulized treatments.

Ⓟ Symptoms of emphysema include mild dyspnea on exertion that progresses to dyspnea at rest as the disease progresses. The patient is usually tachypneic but rarely has a cough.

Ⓟ Bronchiolitis usually starts with signs of an upper respiratory tract infection which progresses to dyspnea, cough, poor feeding, irritability and lethargy.

Ⓟ Patients with a pulmonary emboli may have an accentuated S_2 heart sound.

Ⓟ A flail chest segment is defined as two or more adjacent ribs fractures in two or more locations or detachment of the sternum.

Ⓟ When possible, patients with a pulmonary contusion should be cared for in the semi-Fowler's position to facilitate lung re-expansion.

Ⓟ Air entrapment masks (Venturi masks) must be securely fitted to the face to be effective.

Ⓟ Ataxic respirations are described as an irregular breathing that combines some deep and shallow respirations with periods of apnea.

Ⓟ Ataxic respirations associated with intracranial pressure is a poor indicator for positive patient outcome.

Ⓟ Fremitus is the ability to feel sound waves hit the chest wall during verbalization.

Ⓟ Fremitus is felt over healthy lung tissue, is decreased over areas of obstruction, pneumothorax or emphysema and is increased over areas of consolidation (e.g. pneumonia).

Ⓟ Asthma tends to run in families.

Ⓟ When confirming endotracheal tube placement, epigastric auscultation should precede chest auscultation.

Ⓟ The effects of respiratory or metabolic alkalosis mimic hypocalcemia.

Ⓟ Chronic bronchitis and emphysema can be partially controlled but not cured.

Ⓟ The untoward effects of bronchiolitis are often most severe 24 to 72 hours after the onset of the illness.

Ⓟ Fractures of the sternum are associated with a blunt cardiac injury.

Ⓟ An alternate position for a patient with a pulmonary contusion is side-lying with the injured side up so that gravity will pull blood in the pulmonary vasculature to the lower less affected lung resulting in improved gas exchange.

Ⓟ Patients with tracheobronchial injury will have decreased breath sounds on the affected side.

Ⓟ If vomitus is noted in the mouth or throat of a patient at-risk, suctioning should be emergently instituted as this can remove some or all of the potential aspirate.

Ⓟ The usual place for air leaks when using full face masks in CPAP and BiPAP therapy is either at the bridge of the nose or the corners of the mouth.

- ℗ Right mainstem bronchus intubation is more common then left mainstem bronchus intubation in the adult patient because the right bronchus bifurcates higher on the right.
- ℗ When drawing an arterial blood gas, once the artery is cannulated, the needle should automatically fill with blood unless the patient is significantly hypotensive.
- ℗ Respiratory or metabolic acidosis can include lightheadedness, anxiety, paresthesias (especially the fingers) and circumoral numbness.
- ℗ Never raise a chest drainage system above the level of the chest as this will allow fluid to re-enter the chest and increase the risk of intrapleural infection.
- ℗ Emphysema patients are often tachypneic resulting in normal partial pressures of oxygen and decreased levels of carbon dioxide.
- ℗ Respiratory indications of bronchiolitis include tachypnea (infants may even have periods of apnea), grunting, nasal flaring, intercostal retractions, cyanosis and wheezing on auscultation.

℗ A flail chest results in a free floating segment of the rib cage. The loss of bony structure and resulting pain causes a decrease in respiratory effort.

℗ Elevating the head of the bed to 30 degrees during CPAP and BiPAP therapy minimizes air leaking in the seal of the mask.

℗ The use of combitubes is limited to unconscious patients who have no gag reflex.

℗ Patients on a ventilator with positive end expiratory pressure (PEEP) should be monitored closely for hypotension.

℗ A tension pneumothorax occurs when there is ingress of air into the pleural space without egress of air.

℗ Use of air entrapment masks (Venturi masks) may cause drying of the eyes.

℗ Severe states of alkalosis may cause confusion, tetany, syncope and seizures.

℗ Status asthmaticus causes a pulsus paradoxus.

Ⓟ The amount of blood that can accumulate in the pleural space with a large hemothorax can cause hypovolemia.

Ⓟ Signs of asthma exacerbation include a cough, a sensation of tightness in the chest and wheezing on exhalation that progresses to wheezing on inhalation as the asthma attack progresses.

Ⓟ Additional signs of asthma include crackles, prolonged expiratory time on auscultation, pulsus paradoxus, hyperresonance, restlessness (from hypoxia) and increased work of breathing.

Ⓟ Intubation and mechanical ventilation will be considered for low oxygen saturations associated with large pulmonary contusions.

Ⓟ High frequency noise is transmitted across fluid or abnormal lung tissue more readily than it is transmitted across air. This is referred to as egophany.

Ⓟ Cricoid pressure should be maintained until the trachea has been intubated, the tube position confirmed, and the endotracheal cuff inflated.

- ℗ Albuterol (Proventil, Ventolin) is fairly beta-two specific with less beta-one effects then many other bronchodilators. The effects of this medication lasts 4 -6 hours.
- ℗ Avoid administering nebulizer treatments to a crying child as crying decreases absorption of the medication.
- ℗ Status asthmaticus results in arterial blood gases with hypoxemia, hypercarbia and metabolic acidosis.
- ℗ Over time, the trapping of air in the alveoli caused by emphysema will lead to an increase in the diameter of the chest.
- ℗ When depressing the bulb of an esophageal detector device, immediate re-inflation of the bulb indicates likely tracheal placement, whereas continued deflation indicates esophageal placement.
- ℗ The classic symptom of a flail chest segment is known as paradoxical chest wall movement.
- ℗ The chest x-ray of the child with bronchiolitis may demonstrate signs of air trapping.

℗ Paradoxical chest wall movement is recognized by the flail segment being drawn inward while the rest of the chest expands during inhalation, and the flail segment bulging outwards as the rest of the chest collapses inward during exhalation.

℗ Signs of diaphragmatic rupture include lower chest, abdominal or epigastric pain that radiates to the left shoulder, dyspnea and decreased breath sounds on the affected side.

℗ The head of a patient should be placed in the sniffing position for nasopharyngeal suctioning. Oropharyngeal suctioning can be carried out with the patient's head in any position.

℗ 1 – 2 milliliters of blood is required for an arterial blood gas sample. (0.5 to 1 milliliter in children.)

℗ Never allow the tubing leading from a chest tube to coil below the top of a chest drainage device, as this allows fluid to collect in the dependent loops, increasing pressures within the tubing.

- Ⓟ When air enters the pleural space from an external wound, it is called an open pneumothorax.
- Ⓟ Kinking of the tubing associated with a chest tube will cause intermittent bubbling of water in the water seal chamber to cease. Re-expansion of the pneumothorax may also cause this finding.
- Ⓟ Encourage patients with asthma to encase pillows and mattresses in vinyl and wash bedding every week in water temperatures that exceed 130°F (54.5°C).
- Ⓟ On the chest x-ray of a patient with emphysema, the diaphragm may appear to be pushed down under the hyper-inflated lungs and the heart may appear smaller.
- Ⓟ Aside from chest pain, other indications of pneumonia include tachypnea, tachycardia, and a possible pleural friction rub.
- Ⓟ Common causes of open an open pneumothorax include penetrating trauma to the chest or compound rib fractures.

℗ Air entrapment masks (Venturi masks) deliver oxygen at an FiO_2 of 24%, 28%, 35%, 40% or 50% depending on the aperture of the conduit utilized.

℗ Esophageal detector devices are unreliable in children less than one year of age, morbidly obese patients, and in patients near the end of pregnancy.

℗ Excess acids in the body (aspirin, methanol, paraldehyde) are one cause of metabolic acidosis.

℗ Excess acid production (hyperthyroidism, hypermetabolic states, lactic acidosis, ketogenesis, shock) or impaired acid secretion (acute renal failure, severe hypovolemia, hypoaldosteronism) all contribute to metabolic acidosis.

℗ Excessive losses of bicarbonate (diarrhea, intestinal decompression and draining lower gastrointestinal fistulas) all contribute to metabolic acidosis.

℗ A ruptured diaphragm may cause obstructive shock.

Ⓟ To assess for egophany, auscultate the chest while asking the patient to say the letter "e".

Ⓟ Emphysema typically starts between the ages of 50 and 75 years of age.

Ⓟ When assessing for egophany, areas of fluid or consolidation will cause lower frequencies to be filtered out and "e" will sound more like "a" with the stethoscope.

Ⓟ Positive pressure ventilations dampen fluctuations in the water seal chamber.

Ⓟ Early in the asthma exacerbation, patients tend to have a respiratory alkalosis but as the asthma continues, hypoxia drives a respiratory acidosis.

Ⓟ Patients with asthma should be encouraged to remain inside with air conditioning during the early morning and midday hours.

Ⓟ Heliox (a treatment where nitrogen in air is replaced with helium) may be given to patients with status asthmaticus.

Ⓟ Patients with emphysema often lean forward to breathe and use their accessory muscles to help move their air.

Ⓟ The temperature of a patient with bacterial pneumonia will usually rise faster and higher then with other forms of pneumonia.

Ⓟ Pneumonia is marked by an elevated temperature. (Exceptions include the neonate or the elderly who can have subnormal temperatures associated with pneumonia).

Ⓟ A large pulmonary emboli may cause signs of right sided heart failure and profound hypotension.

Ⓟ In adults, foreign objects are more likely to lodge in the right bronchi because of its lesser angle of convergence. In pediatric patients, there is no difference between obstruction in the right and left bronchi.

Ⓟ Aside from paradoxical chest wall movement, other signs of a flail chest include pain, increased respiratory effort, decreased tidal volume, impaired cough and hypoxia.

Ⓟ The use of high concentrations of oxygen may cause collapse of the alveoli and production of oxygen waste products, leading to worsening rather than improving respiratory status, therefore, the FiO_2 of delivered oxygen should only be as high as required to keep saturations above 90%.

Ⓟ When using a bag-mask device, compression of the bag should occur over one second.

Ⓟ Ventilation of the stomach is easier than ventilation of the lungs, therefore, lack of bag compliance when using a bag-mask device following intubation may be an indication of esophageal intubation.

Ⓟ A serum pH below 7.2 will cause symptoms such as Kussmaul's respirations, dysrhythmias and CNS depression (confusion, drowsiness, lethargy, stupor, coma).

Ⓟ Patients in status asthmaticus often require intubation so that drugs can be delivered deeper into the lungs via the endotracheal tube.

Ⓟ 80 – 90% of aspirated objects lodge in the bronchi.

Ⓟ A classic sign of emphysema is pursed lip breathing. Other findings include hyperresonance on percussion and speaking in short sentences to reduce breathlessness.

Ⓟ Pleuritic chest pain is common with pneumonia. It may be referred diaphragmatically and be mistaken for abdominal illnesses.

Ⓟ Symptoms of pulmonary edema include orthopnea/dyspnea, tachypnea leading to respiratory alkalosis, hypoxia that may lead to metabolic acidosis and cardiac dysrhythmias, crackles and wheezes on auscultation and frothy/blood-tinged sputum.

Ⓟ One symptom found with fat emboli not found with other forms of pulmonary emboli is petechiae of the chest, conjunctiva and axilla.

Ⓟ Injuries associated with flail chests include pulmonary contusions, a hemothorax or pneumothorax and blunt cardiac injuries.

Ⓟ Bowel sounds may be auscultated in the chest if a patient has a ruptured diaphragm.

- Ⓟ For nasopharyngeal suctioning, the diameter of the suction catheter should be no more than one half of the diameter of the nares to be suctioned.
- Ⓟ A serum pH below 7.0 will result in bradycardia.
- Ⓟ Excessive volumes when using a bag-mask device can cause a pneumothorax or gastric insufflation.
- Ⓟ Condensation on the inside of the endotracheal tube during exhalation is an indicator of proper tube placement.
- Ⓟ Central neurogenic hyperventilation is a respiratory pattern with deep, rapid respirations without apneic periods associated with increased intracranial pressure.
- Ⓟ Signs of increased intrathoracic pressure include the presence of jugular venous distension.
- Ⓟ Apply direct pressure to an arterial blood gas site for a minimum of 3 to 5 minutes. (10 minutes if the patient is on anticoagulants).

Ⓟ Conditions which can cause metabolic alkalosis include vomiting, gastric suction and diuretic therapy.

Ⓟ When the kidneys conserve positive ions (potassium-sparing diuretics, hypokalemia states and hypomagnesemia states), patients develop metabolic alkalosis.

Ⓟ Excessive bicarbonate in the body (excessive intravenous bicarbonate or excess baking soda used as a home remedy) contribute to metabolic alkalosis.

Ⓟ Fluid in the pleural space commonly causes a dull ache low in the chest on the affected side. A pneumothorax causes a sharp pain on inspiration near the shoulder on the affected side.

Ⓟ Percussion over fluid in the pleural space will cause hyporesonance, percussion over air in the pneumothorax will cause hyperresonance.

Ⓟ Teach patients with asthma to keep cats and dogs outside the house and to consider carpet removal and antimite treatment.

Ⓟ Kussmaul's respirations are associated with acidosis.

Ⓟ Kussmaul's respirations are defined as regular, deep, and labored respirations.

Ⓟ Continuous bubbling in a chest drainage system when the system is patent may be an indication of a bronchial tear.

Ⓟ If continuous bubbling exists in the water seal chamber of a chest drainage system, make sure all tubing connections are tight, applying tape to connections as appropriate. If the continuous bubbling continues in the water seal chamber, apply or re-inforce the occlusive dressing at the chest tube insertion site. If continuous bubbling continues at this point in the water seal chamber of a chest drainage system, consider changing out the tubing and chest drainage system.

Ⓟ Isoetherine (Bronkosol, Bronkometer) is a very beta-two specific bronchodilator with minimal beta-one effects. It has a rapid onset of action but the duration of effects is short.

- Ⓟ If the patient is already hypoxic when intubation is performed, monitor closely for hypoxic ventricular dysrhythmias during intubation.
- Ⓟ Treatment for emphysema and chronic bronchitis exacerbations may include CPAP, BiPAP, beta-adrenergic agonists, mucolytics, anti-inflammatory drugs and steroids.
- Ⓟ The cough of bacterial pneumonia may be productive for purulent material.
- Ⓟ One treatment goal for pulmonary edema is to improve oxygenation through administration of high flow oxygen, BiPAP , CPAP or intubation and mechanical ventilation.
- Ⓟ Diagnosis of pulmonary emboli may be made with a lung scan, high-resolution helical computed tomographic angiography, V/Q scans or pulmonary angiography.
- Ⓟ Two main concerns associated with fractures of the ribs are pain management and prevention of respiratory complications.

Ⓟ When using non-rebreather masks, the reservoir must be filled before applying the mask to the patient.

Ⓟ The endotracheal tube should be visualized just above the carina on chest x-ray if it is properly positioned.

Ⓟ If intercostal muscle retractions are localized to one area of the chest, suspect obstruction in the large bronchi.

Ⓟ A low serum pH, high carbon dioxide level and normal bicarbonate level is associated with respiratory acidosis.

Ⓟ A high serum pH with an increased carbon dioxide level and normal bicarbonate level is associated with respiratory alkalosis.

Ⓟ A low serum pH, normal carbon dioxide level and decreased bicarbonate level is associated with metabolic acidosis.

Ⓟ An increased serum pH with a normal carbon dioxide level and an increased bicarbonate level is associated with metabolic alkalosis.

Ⓟ Heart sounds may shift to the right in patients with a ruptured diaphragm.

- Ⓟ Asthma causes breath sounds to diminish in the lower lobes first, and decrease upwards as the asthma attack progresses.
- Ⓟ Always institute cardiac monitoring on patients with chronic obstructive pulmonary disease because they are at risk of hypoxic dysrhythmias.
- Ⓟ Combitubes should not be used on patient's under five feet tall.
- Ⓟ When assessing over the area of pneumonia, decreased breath sounds, hyporesonance to percussion and increased fremitus may be noted.
- Ⓟ The blood gases of a patient with a pulmonary emboli may demonstrate decreased oxygen pressure and decreased pCO_2.
- Ⓟ Pain management is a goal in the patient with rib fractures, not only for comfort, but also to allow the patient to participate in incentive spirometry to prevent respiratory complications.
- Ⓟ Pain management in patients with respiratory emergencies should not blunt the respiratory drive, which can increase the risk for pulmonary infections.

Ⓟ Some patients with rib fractures may require intercostal nerve blocks for pain relief.

Ⓟ The reservoir bag of a non-rebreather mask should not deflate, even with deep inspiration. If this occurs, the oxygen flow should be increased to prevent re-breathing of carbon dioxide.

Ⓟ When ventilating a patient in cardiac arrest with a bag-mask device, 8 to 10 breaths per minute should be delivered.

Ⓟ When ventilating an adult patient with a pulse using a bag-mask device, 10 - 12 breaths per minute should be delivered.

Ⓟ When ventilating a pediatric patient with a pulse, using a bag-mask device, 12 - 20 breaths per minute should be delivered.

Ⓟ Disposable colorometric carbon dioxide detector devices turn yellow when exposed to carbon dioxide and are blue or purple in the presence of oxygen.

Ⓟ When using beta-two agonists inhalers, patients should be encouraged to wait one minute between puffs.

Ⓟ The ventilator should be set with small tidal volumes on patients with status asthmaticus who have been intubated.

Ⓟ Expel all gas bubbles from the needle after an arterial blood gas sample has been obtained or the partial pressure of oxygen may be falsely elevated.

Ⓟ A compensating metabolic acidosis results in a low pH, low bicarbonate level and low carbon dioxide level.

Ⓟ A compensating respiratory acidosis results in a low pH, high bicarbonate level and high carbon dioxide level.

Ⓟ A compensating metabolic alkalosis results in a high pH, high bicarbonate level and high carbon dioxide level.

Ⓟ A compensating respiratory alkalosis results in a high pH, low bicarbonate level and low carbon dioxide level.

Ⓟ In order for air to be drawn into the chest with an open pneumothorax, the opening must be larger than 2/3 the diameter of the trachea.

Ⓟ If a patient vomits while cricoid pressure is applied, the pressure should be released to prevent esophageal rupture.

Ⓟ Elderly patients with pneumonia may present with nothing more than a change in sensorium.

Ⓟ Allow patients with chronic obstructive pulmonary disease to assume a position of comfort which is often sitting up and leaning forward.

Ⓟ Because bronchitis is viral, supportive therapies such as administration of cough preparations for sleep, humidification to loosen secretions, bronchodilators and corticosteroids are utilized.

Ⓟ Indications for admitting a child with bronchiolitis includes signs of respiratory fatigue, oxygen saturations less than 90%, respiratory rates above 70 breaths per minute and apneic episodes.

Ⓟ Complete obstructions of the upper airway require the Heimlich maneuver. This maneuver should not be performed on patients with partial obstructions (coughing, gagging or verbalizing).

Ⓟ Apnea is used to describe lack of respirations.

Ⓟ To use a bulb suction on infants, the bulb should be depressed before inserting it into the mouth and nose and released when it is in the area of secretions.

Ⓟ Cheyne-Stoke respirations signify a build-up of carbon dioxide in the cerebrum.

Ⓟ Make sure the side ports of oxygen face masks do not become blocked. This can lead to re-breathing of carbon dioxide.

Ⓟ When using end-tidal CO_2 colorimetric devices, remember that "gold is good" (gold on exhalation indicates the presence of CO_2, a strong indicator that the tube is in the trachea).

Ⓟ When using end-tidal CO_2 colorimetric devices remember "**Y**ellow means **Y**es" and "**P**urple means **P**oor".

Ⓟ To ventilate a needle cricothyrotomy using a bag-mask device, place a 3.0 endotracheal tube adaptor over the needle or cricothyrotomy device then attach the bag device to the adaptor.

Ⓟ Cheyne-Stoke respirations are a pattern of breathing with a rhythmic crescendo and decrescendo of the rate and depth of respiration punctuated by brief periods of apnea.

Ⓟ Generalized intercostal muscle retractions are indicative of diseases such as emphysema, asthma, or chronic bronchitis.

Ⓟ To relieve a tension pneumothorax emergently, insert a 1.2 – 2.4 inch (3 to 6 centimeter) long 10 to 16 gauge over the needle catheter into the pleural space.

Ⓟ Salmeterol zinaoate (Serevent) has a long onset of action and long duration of action, therefore, it is not useful for acute exacerbation of asthma, but may be used for control of symptoms.

Ⓟ When using a metered dose inhaler, tell the patient to shake the inhaler and hold it one to two inches from the face before taking a puff. Then exhale, press on the puffer, inhale deeply and hold the breath for a count of ten.

ⓅAfter drawing blood for an arterial blood gas sample, rotate the syringe to mix the heparin with the blood.

ⓅAn open pneumothorax causes a sucking sound during inspiration if the patient is breathing spontaneously. If a patient is intubated, the wound over an open pneumothorax will bubble when the bag-mask device is compressed.

ⓅThe directions for a spacer are the same as for a metered dose inhaler, except the patient should press on the inhaler and wait five seconds before inhaling.

ⓅFremitus is absent when there is fluid in the pleural space. Fremitus may be present but decreased over a pneumothorax.

ⓅDevelopment of a pneumothorax after intubation is a risk factor when intubating a patient in status asthmaticus.

ⓅPresenting symptoms of children with pneumonia may include a nonproductive cough, grunting, intercostal muscle retractions, vomiting, poor feeding and fatigue.

Ⓟ Apneustic breathing is marked by prolonged inspiratory and expiratory pauses of 2 to 3 seconds. This respiratory pattern is consis-
tent with brainstem lesions at the level of the pons.

Ⓟ It is essential to stress the importance of pneumococcal and viral
immunizations in patients with chronic obstructive pulmonary disease because they are at high risk of pulmonary infections.

Ⓟ Patients with pulmonary edema should be encouraged to sit upright with the legs dangling if they can tolerate that position to
allow pooling of blood in the lower extremities.

Ⓟ Laboratory tests associated with pulmonary emboli may show an
elevated erythrocyte sedimentation rate (ESR), and increased fi-
brin-split products, especially an elevated D-Dimer.

Ⓟ To prevent pulmonary complications, patients with rib fractures
need to be taught how to perform deep breathing and coughing
exercises as well as incentive spirometry.

Ⓟ A patient with a partial obstruction will usually undergo endoscopic removal of the object.

Ⓟ Encourage patients with chronic obstructive pulmonary disease to stay adequately hydrated, exercise regularly and to stop smoking.

Ⓟ If an endotracheal tube is correctly placed, no sounds should be auscultated over the epigastrium and breath sounds should be easily heard over the right and left lung fields after intubation.

Ⓟ Tracheobronchial injuries associated with severe air leaks and significant respiratory distress may require immediate intubation with the tube being placed below the level of the injury.

Ⓟ Patients with rib fractures will usually require oxygen administration until pain control is achieved to overcome respiratory splinting.

Ⓟ The white blood cell count is usually higher in a patient with bacterial pneumonia then a patient with other forms of pneumonia.

Ⓟ Encourage patients with chronic obstructive pulmonary disease to avoid crowds and situations in which there is a high likelihood of exposure to respiratory infections.

Ⓟ For oral suctioning with a bulb suction, the tip should be applied to the side pockets of the cheeks, but not to the back of the throat.

Ⓟ Tracheobronchial injuries may have subcutaneous emphysema to the chest, neck and face as well as a continuous air leak in the chest drainage unit.

Ⓟ Children may be more compliant with oxygen therapy if they are allowed to handle the cannula or mask before it is applied.

Ⓟ In cases of multiple rib fractures or a flail chest, mechanical intubation with positive end expiratory pressure or even internal fixation of the ribs with screws and plates may be required.

Ⓟ Because crying can cause an airway obstruction to shift, children with suspected or known airway obstructions should be carefully managed to avoid or minimize crying.

- Ⓟ The electrocardiogram of a patient with pulmonary emboli may show a new onset right bundle branch block and right axis deviation with peaked P waves in the limb leads as well as depressed T waves in the right precordial leads.

- Ⓟ Treatment for bronchiolitis includes oxygen administration, antivirals, anticholinergics, and adrenergic stimulants.

- Ⓟ Patients with chronic obstructive pulmonary disease should be encouraged to eat small, frequent meals to allow maximal excursion of the chest.

- Ⓟ If pressures applied with CPAP or BiPAP exceed 20 cm of water, a gastric tube should be considered to prevent gastric distension.

- Ⓟ Recent ingestion of carbonated beverages or antacids may cause a false positive result when using a disposable colorometric carbon dioxide detector device. (This effect is generally nullified after six compressions of the bag-mask device.)

Ⓟ Needle cricothyrotomies do not allow for adequate release of carbon dioxide and should be reserved for short term use.

Ⓟ Diaphragmatic breathing is an indicator of respiratory distress in the adult patient but is a normal finding in the pediatric patient.

Ⓟ A drop of more than 10 mm Hg between the systolic blood pressure at the height of inhalation and the systolic blood pressure during exhalation is known as pulsus paradoxus.

Ⓟ Accessory muscle use is an indicator of respiratory distress in adult patients but is less likely to be noted in the pediatric population because these muscles are underdeveloped in the young.

Ⓟ Pulsus paradoxus is an indicator of increased intrathoracic pressure.

Ⓟ A tension pneumothorax puts pressure on the unaffected lung, the heart and the great vessels causing obstructive shock.

Ⓟ A patient with a normal serum pH, but an abnormal bicarbonate and carbon dioxide level has a fully compensated blood gas.

Ⓟ If the pH is below 7.40 in a fully compensated blood gas, the patient is recovering from acidosis, if the pH is above 7.40 in a fully compensated blood gas, the patient is recovering from an alkalosis.

Ⓟ When relieving a tension pneumothorax by inserting a needle, the needle should be placed above the third rib in the second intercostal space at the midclavicular line.

Ⓟ An elevated temperature can increase the partial pressure of oxygen in an arterial blood gas sample. Document a patient's temperature when transporting an arterial blood gas sample.

Ⓟ Egophany will be noted over fluid accumulations in the pleural space, but not over air accumulations.

Ⓟ Signs of a tension pneumothorax include severe respiratory distress, chest pain, decreased or absent breath sounds on the affected side, signs of obstructive shock, jugular venous distension and tracheal deviation away from the pneumothorax.

Ⓟ Severe hypoxia in children may cause somnolence, decreased respiratory effort, bradycardia and even periodic apnea.

Ⓟ Xopenex (Levabuterol) is a bronchodilator with rapid onset of action that causes specific beta-two effects and minimal beta-one effects.

Ⓟ When ventilating a patient with asthma who has been intubated, only compress the bag until resistance is felt to prevent a pneumothorax.

Ⓟ Patients at risk for aspiration need to be thoughtfully positioned with either their head elevated or in a side-lying position to decrease their risk.

Ⓟ Bronchiolitis is usually diagnosed via a nasopharyngeal culture.

Ⓟ Short-term oxygen therapy should not be withheld from patients with chronic obstructive pulmonary disease. Enough oxygen should be given to maintain the patient's normal oxygen saturation level.

- ℗ After placing the needle in the pleural space for a tension pneumothorax, there should be a rush of air from the needle and the patient's respiratory status should improve immediately.
- ℗ Generally, an oxygen saturation of 90 to 92% is desirable for COPD patients.
- ℗ If children are to be discharged with bronchiolitis, teach parents how to do home nebulizer treatments and encourage small frequent feedings to keep the diaphragm low.
- ℗ Morphine and nitroglycerin (Nitrostat) may be administered for their vasodilatory properties to patients with pulmonary edema.
- ℗ Equipment for performance of a surgical airway, such as a cricothyrotomy or tracheostomy, should be readily available if a partial airway obstruction is high in the airway.
- ℗ End tidal carbon dioxide detectors may be inaccurate when used during cardiac arrest because insufficient carbon dioxide is not circulated to the lungs.

Ⓟ When suctioning a patient, administer supplemental oxygen between each passage of the suction catheter.

Ⓟ Ipratropium (Atrovent) is a parasympatholytic with anticholinergic side effects such as dry mouth and eyes, pupil dilation, and blurred vision. It is used to prevent bronchoconstriction in asthma.

Ⓟ When teaching a patient to do peak expiratory flow rates at home, a reading that is 50 – 79% of normal should result in inhaler use, a reading of less than 50% of normal should result in the patient seeking medical attention.

Ⓟ An abnormal decrease in respiratory rates may be an indication of the need to reduce oxygen therapy in the patient with chronic obstructive pulmonary disease.

Ⓟ Furosemide (to decrease intravascular volume), digoxin (to improve cardiac contractibility), dopamine (to increase blood pressure) and nitropress (to decrease afterload) are all considered in the treatment of pulmonary edema.

Ⓟ If a patient can tolerate the position and the injuries do not contra-indicate it, consider nursing a patient with a flail chest segment with the injured side down against the bed.

Ⓟ Patients with a ruptured diaphragm should receive supplemental oxygen, an intravenous line, treatment for hypovolemic shock and transfer to the surgical suite for repair of the injury.

Ⓟ Children may be more compliant if the parent is allowed to hold the oxygen delivery apparatus up to or near the child's face.

Ⓟ It is essential to use pediatric sized end-tidal carbon dioxide detectors to prevent removing too many gases from the ventilation.

Ⓟ Monitor for a pneumothorax or hypotension when caring for patients on CPAP and BiPAP therapy.

Ⓟ If the tubing of a chest drainage system becomes dislodged from the chest drainage system, immediately submerge the exposed tubing into 0.8 to 1.0 inches (2 to 2.5 centimeters) of sterile water.

Ⓟ Decreased breath sounds, oxygen saturations, respiratory effort and levels of consciousness are indications of impending respiratory failure that will require emergent intervention.

Ⓟ Antibiotic administration within four hours of arrival in the ED should be the goal in patients who present with bacterial pneumonia.

Ⓟ Treatment for pulmonary emboli includes high flow oxygen administration, intravenous fluids or vasopressors for hypotension, and anticoagulants or fibrinolytic agents.

Ⓟ Most patients with a tracheobronchial injury will have better respiratory status in the upright position.

Ⓟ Pediatric sized combitubes are not available; therefore combitubes should not be used on this age group.

Ⓟ When assessing for endotracheal tube placement on the pediatric patient, auscultate at the midaxillary lines rather than the midclavicular lines to assess for breath sounds.

- Ⓟ Pediatric patients are especially susceptible to gastric insufflation when ventilating them with a bag-mask device; therefore, early passage of a gastric tube should be considered.
- Ⓟ Transport arterial blood gas samples on ice.
- Ⓟ Needle cricothyrotomies are the preferred method of surgical airway management in children under the age of 12.
- Ⓟ Crackles on auscultation are produced by the movement of air through secretions or lightly closed airways.

Bibliography for respiratory emergencies

American College of Surgeons Committee on Trauma. (2002). *Management of the airway*. Retrieved December 24, 2011, from American College of Surgeons: http://www.facs.org/trauma/publications/airway.pdf

American Heart Association. (2005). *Circulation 112 (Supplement IV)*. Retrieved January 1, 2009, from American Heart Association guidelines for cardiopulmonary resuscitation and emergency cardiovascular care: http://circ.ahajournals.org/content/vol112/issue4/

Dave, A. (2002). Absent Nasal Flaring in a Newborn With Bilateral Choanal Stenosis. *Pediatrics , 109* (5), 989-990.

Elsevier Mosby. (2005). *Mosby's Expert 10-minute physical examination.* St. Louis: Elsevier Mosby.

Emergency Nurses Association. (2004). *Emergency Nursing Pediatric Course Provider Manual* (3 ed.). Des Plaines: Emergency Nurses Association.

Emergency Nurses Association. (2007). *Trauma Nursing Core Course Provider Manual* (6 ed.). Des Plaines Il: Emergency Nurses Association.

Hammond, BB. Gerber-Zimmerman, P. (Ed.). (2013). *Sheehy's manual of emergency care* (7 ed.). St. Louis: Mosby.

Hedges, J. R., Baker, W. E., Laniox, R., & Field, D. L. (2012). Devices for Assessing Oxygenation and Ventilation. In J. R. Roberts, & J. R. Hedges (Eds.), *Clinical procedures in emergency medicine* (5 ed., pp. 22—36). Philadelphia: Saunders.

High, K. (2005). *Airway management.* (D. York-Clark, J. Stocking, & J. Johnson, Eds.) Denver Colorado: Air and surface transport nurses association.

Hoyt, K. S., & Selfridge-Thomas, J. (Eds.). (2007). *Emergency Nursing Core Curriculum* (6 ed.). St. Louis: Saunders Elsevier.

Kunz Howard P, Steinmann, RA. (Eds.) (2010) Sheehy's Emergency Nursing: Principles and Practice. 6th ed. St. Louis: Mosby.

Madappa, T. (2011, September 1). *Pulmonary Disease and Pregnancy*. Retrieved December 24, 2011, from emedicine: http:// emedicine.medscape.com/article/303852-overview

McMahon, M. D. (2009). End-Tidal carbon dioxide detection and monitoring. In J. Proehl, *Emergency nursing procedures* (4 ed., pp. 98 - 104). St. Louis: Saunders-Elsevier.

Murray, A. D. (2011, August 9). *Foreign Bodies of the Airway*. Retrieved December 24, 2011, from emedicine: http://

emedicine.medscape.com/article/872498-overview

Proehl, J. (2009). *Emergency Nursing Procedures* (4 ed.). St. Louis: Saunders.